Unexpected

Everything They Don't Tell You About Pregnancy,
Childbirth, and Life With a Newborn

Lindsey Barton

D1712975

Table of Contents

Forward

Hey Mama! Welcome to the hardest, messiest, and most rewarding time of your life. Whether you just found out you're expecting, are about to give birth, or you're just trying to figure out life with a newborn… this book is for you. I may just be your average stay-at-home mom but when you mix in OCD and anxiety… BAM! You have the perfect neurotic mom friend to tell you all the stuff no one talks about. Trust me when I say I have researched it all and I have been through most of it! While Google saved me numerous times the past few years, a lot of what I have learned came straight from my mom intuition, something we all instinctually have!

I am not a nutritionist, I am not a financial advisor, and I am certainly not a childcare expert. I am, however, a mom who wants to raise a healthy, happy baby and share what I have learned with other moms, like you.

With my first and only baby, I had no idea what to expect (despite reading "What to Expect When You're Expecting" twice). Everything was new and scary, and I felt so overwhelmed. Maybe you feel that way too? If so, you're in the right place. I had to figure all of this out on my own, since most of the stuff in this book isn't talked about much, if at all. I did the hard work for you, so you can focus on yourself and your baby! What are friends for, right?

I'll be the first to admit, raising kids is hard! I really don't understand how our parents managed raising us without being able to Google every runny nose or hop on Pinterest for last minute Crock-Pot recipes. But somehow, they did! I mean, we're still alive, aren't we? They survived, and you will too!

There's a Baby in There!?

I'm going to share something with you that will either make you think, *oh my gosh me too!* or it will make you think I'm crazy. Seriously, I can feel the eye rolls already. I knew almost instantly that I was pregnant. It's hard to explain unless you've felt the same way, but my body was different so fast that I even told my sister in law two weeks later that I was pretty sure I was pregnant. I hadn't missed a period and I wasn't experiencing any of the early pregnancy symptoms yet…but it was enough to call bs on all the women on that show who didn't know they were pregnant until they were in labor. I mean, how could they not know!? I didn't know for sure because I hadn't taken a test yet, and I was in a little bit of denial, but subconsciously I knew.

The Test!

I always pictured myself finding out I was pregnant by taking a pregnancy test, pacing around the bathroom awaiting the results, seeing the two pink lines and being overwhelmed with joy. But that wasn't how it happened for me since my daughter wasn't planned. I decided to take a home pregnancy test, so after work one day I drove 15 minutes out of my way to a random Walgreens where the pharmacist didn't know me. Why I was acting like a teenager buying condoms, I'm not sure, but I didn't want anyone to notice me. I kept my sunglasses on, grabbed the cheapest test, and headed to the register. I felt like everyone around me was staring at me, even though I'm sure they couldn't care less. I was 25 years old, so I don't know why I was so embarrassed about buying a pregnancy test, but I was. Now, obviously if you are trying to get pregnant you could always go to your doctor for a blood test because that will be the most accurate way to know for sure. But for me, I just needed to know what was going on (and to see if I actually was crazy).

I was under the impression that I had to WAIT a few minutes to find out the results of a pregnancy test. I mean, the instructions said to pee on the stick, or pee in a cup and set the stick in said pee, and then lay it down for a few minutes while the results come in. The first thing no one told me...brace yourself because sometimes those pink lines show up immediately. If you are trying to get pregnant, then this could be great news! But as for me, I was so not prepared. I no sooner sat down and started going when those two pink lines instantly showed up. *What in the actual hell?* I thought to myself. That should have been my first warning that this baby would definitely make her presence known in this world. I recommend you at least hold onto a wall or something because you might pass out if you stare at the test like I did. Not only did those two pink lines show up right away, but I also went into shock and almost blacked out on the toilet. *Get it together,* I thought to myself, *your baby's dad cannot find out you're pregnant by walking in on you sprawled out on the bathroom floor with your butt in the air and a pregnancy test in your hand.*

So, What Now?

So many things were running through my head that I sat on the toilet for another few minutes staring at the test. Once I got up, my legs were shaking, and I began pacing around the bathroom. This was really happening. There is an actual person taking up residency inside of my uterus. I don't know how to explain the feeling of knowing you are pregnant for the first time because I am sure it is different for every woman depending on where she's at in life. I felt like I was in a dream and everything felt surreal. Forgetting for a split second that I wasn't the first woman in the world to get pregnant I decided to call my OB. She's been my doctor since I was 16 and literally knows me inside and out so of course she would know what to do! I may be the only person who called her lady doctor before her partner or her mother when she found out she was pregnant, but again it's not like I planned this. My doctor was thrilled and told me to come see her in five weeks. *Five weeks!?* I thought, *what on earth am I supposed to do with this thing for five weeks?* I made the appointment anyways and sat on the couch trying to wrap my head around everything.

Sharing the News

I spent years picturing this exact moment and what it would be like and it was finally here. My next step? I did what every girl in her mid-twenties would do in a situation like this…I logged onto Pinterest for help. As I searched for cute ways to tell people I was pregnant, I began to get excited for the first time since this all started less than an hour before. I don't know if your pregnancy was planned or not, but I just want to say that no matter how your baby comes to be, I fully believe they are here for a reason and are a blessing from above. I hadn't planned on my daughter, but she was in there, and I wanted to make the best of it.

I landed on a cute idea to tell Will, the dad-to-be, and headed to the motherland…Target. Still shaking, I walked towards the baby section, a place I had only been once before when my brother and sister-in-law were having my niece. To be honest, this section of Target always gave me massive anxiety. There were always babies crying and moms trying to buy diapers with kids hanging off her…I was always afraid I would run over a stray child with my cart by accident if I got too close. As I approached this newfound territory, it was surprisingly quiet. I watched the other moms with their babies and had to fight the urge to shout out, *hey! I'm one of you guys now!* Because that would be weird, right? I (quietly) browsed all the different baby things and got a little nervous when I realized how much stuff this kid would actually need.

By the way, it is totally normal to feel overwhelmed at this point, and I had to keep reminding myself of this every time I turned a corner and more baby stuff smacked me in the face. I found a little blue and white long sleeve onesie that said "I Love Daddy" on it and threw it in my cart. I was so nervous about how he would react that I chose blue instead of pink. For some dumb reason I thought he would be more excited if he thought the baby was a boy, even though it was only the size of a sesame seed at this point. It was weird, I know. I grabbed a red gift bag and some white tissue paper (had to stop myself from grabbing a few bottles of wine) and checked out. I placed the gift bag on the kitchen table and waited for him to come home. When he got home, he opened the bag and asked if I was serious. *No dummy I thought it would be funny to pretend to be knocked up...of course I'm serious!* I thought, but since I couldn't speak I just nodded. I think he was more excited than I was because he gave me the biggest hug while I sat there and ugly cried. P.S. ugly crying will happen a lot... just embrace it.

The "This Sucks" Trimester

Your first trimester lasts from week 1 to the end of week 12. During this time, most women feel their worst. I was lucky enough to have a pretty easy first trimester. I never threw up, but I did get nauseous quite often and even passed out in my bathroom once. I was blow drying my hair, started to see spots, was smart enough to sit down on the tile, and ended up blacking out. I have no idea how long I was out for, but I remember coming to and for a minute thought I had taken a nap. When I realized I was on my bathroom floor, panic set in. I was home alone and immediately called my sister in law who was a nurse. She rushed over, took one look at me and said, "either you're really dehydrated or you're pregnant". I hadn't planned on telling her this way, but as I have learned this whole pregnancy and raising babies thing laughs in your face every time you try to "plan" anything.

Luckily, that never happened again although I did get close quite a few times. Every woman will experience pregnancy in a totally different way, so there is no rule book on how to survive it. Some women are sick the whole 40 weeks, while others never even get a headache. But, I am here to share what worked for me in hopes that it will help you too!

My First Trimester Essentials

To combat my dizziness, morning (afternoon, and evening) sickness, and to be as comfortable as possible in general, I relied on these things my entire first trimester:

Ginger Lemon Tea
Peppermints and Peppermint Tea
Gummy Prenatal Vitamins
Fruit (mainly peaches and bananas)
Saltines
Leggings
Pregnancy Pillow
WATER
Pregnancy Tracker App
Pregnancy Journal and Scrapbook

1. Tea was a staple item throughout my pregnancy, postpartum, and during nursing. Trust me, Mother Nature knows what she's doing! There are a bunch of different teas out there and some are even designed to help pregnant and nursing moms with a variety of needs. For my first trimester, ginger lemon tea was a life saver. Ginger and lemon work together to ease your nausea and settle your tummy, so it's perfect for that yucky morning sickness. Always check the ingredients list for tea because sometimes there are added sugars, caffeine, and artificial flavoring. Go for the all-natural teas no matter what stage of motherhood you're in and be sure to check that the type of tea you are purchasing is safe for your baby too.

2. Peppermint is amazing for headaches, which can strike at any time during your pregnancy. According to Americanpregnancy.org, during the first trimester

your body experiences a surge of hormones and an increase in blood volume which leads to an increase in headaches. Sipping on peppermint tea, sucking on peppermints, or even just smelling peppermint can offer some much needed relief.

3. Vitamins are an essential part of any daily routine, but as soon as you find out you're expecting you should start taking a prenatal vitamin. No one ever told me that most of them are horse pills that gag you half to death, so I'll let you in on a little secret…gummy vitamins are the way to go! I took the VitaFusion ones and loved them. Morning sickness is bad enough so don't torture yourself by trying to swallow a giant pill and make it worse. Beware though, not all gummy vitamins are created equal. Avoid artificial colors and flavors and check for added sugar before deciding on which brand you want to go with.

4. Fruits. I heard somewhere that when you are pregnant with a girl, you crave sweet stuff and when you're pregnant with a boy, you crave salty stuff. Who knows if that's true or not, but fruit was something that I craved throughout my entire pregnancy (along with other sweet things) with my daughter. Fruit should be a part of your diet no matter what, but it can be especially beneficial during the first trimester. Every time I felt like I was going to faint, I grabbed a peach or a banana. Fruit will give you a natural energy boost and can help regulate your blood sugar, so stock up and munch on it as much as you can.

5. Saltines are probably an obvious one for nausea, but they're worth mentioning. Keeping saltines next to

your bed and in your purse will make them easily accessible if you start feeling weak or nauseous. Don't worry, you purse will turn into a snack bar once your baby starts eating solid foods anyways so it's good to get used to it now. They have healthier versions different from the original Saltines, so check out the organic brands such as Annie's and Back to Nature.

6. Leggings…wonderful, heavenly leggings. Leggings are basically all I wear now and if you don't already have them, you will want to get them! I don't know about you, but when I feel queasy the last thing I want is to be wearing jeans or uncomfortable clothes that press against my belly. I wore them a ton because they're stretchy, super comfy, and they help hide your belly when you're in that awkward "is she getting fat or is she pregnant" phase. Maternity leggings are the bomb because you can wear them after you give birth as well! Something no one ever told me is that you will still look half way pregnant for a while after you give birth, (unless you're a Kardashian) and maternity leggings are prefect for this. The high-waisted stretchy band is great for C section mamas too! Even after you get your pre-baby body back (which you will, I promise), leggings are a great way to look put together and be comfortable while taking care of a baby. Not to mention when your kiddo is a toddler and you're chasing them around, leggings are a Godsend.

7. Pregnancy pillows will help you survive your first, second, and third trimesters so investing in one early is encouraged. Getting comfortable during pregnancy in general is tough, and these pillows are

designed specifically for expecting moms. I purchased the Snoogle, which was a C-shaped one, but they have a bunch out there based off the type of sleeper you are. I learned that when you're pregnant, and especially when you're about to pop, the way you sleep really matters! The best way to sleep is on your left side. Sleeping on your left side increases the amount of blood and nutrients that reach the placenta and your baby. The right side is totally safe too, but left is best! Side sleeping can also help if you're experiencing shortness of breath, which I definitely did. Try to avoid sleeping on your back as this can cause increased backaches, trouble breathing, distress to your digestive system, hemorrhoids (eew), low blood pressure and can cause a decrease in circulation to your heart and your baby. You should also avoid stomach sleeping at all costs because, well duh…there's a baby in there. The full body pillows offer the support you need and are worth every penny. You can also get super soft pillow cases for them!

8. Water is another obvious one, but when you don't feel good, drinking water may not be a priority. I found that investing in a pretty tumbler made me want to drink more water. It also makes it easier to travel with because tumblers keep your drinks colder for long periods of time. Find one you like and fill it with ice water to sip on throughout the day. When your body is working overtime trying to grow a human, you need to stay hydrated!

9. When I found out I was pregnant, one of the first things I did was download a pregnancy tracker app on my phone. This allowed me to see how big my baby was, and it told me what to expect each week.

It also had me take pictures of my bump which was so fun to look back on! There are a few different apps to choose from so test them out and see which one you like best.

10. Finally, get yourself a pregnancy journal or start a scrapbook so you can document everything. It all goes by so quickly and you will most likely want to look back on it someday. Pregnancy journals guide you through the process and ask you to write down milestones, how you're feeling, what you're craving and much more! Some even have a place for you to write notes to your baby. I didn't know about the journals when I was pregnant (if I had you better believe I would have been all over them), but I've always been a scrapbooker so of course I started one right away. Documenting this experience is something you will never regret doing and how cool to think your growing baby will see it one day too? Also, scrapbooking can be very relaxing so go ahead and take all the pictures, buy all the pretty scrapbook paper, and go nuts!

More Tips and Tricks

1. Stay active. I did yoga almost every day (until I was too big and uncomfortable). YouTube has a lot of yoga and exercise videos for pregnant women that you can do at home.

2. Avoid spicy, fatty, or greasy foods…at least for the first trimester! I'm not here to tell you I ate perfectly healthy my entire pregnancy, but until you get past morning sickness…try to avoid these types

of foods and stick to cold or bland foods that will be easy on your tummy.

3. Get out of bed SLOWLY. I cannot tell you how many times I almost went down from getting up too fast, especially in the morning. Take your time, stretch, roll onto your side, sit up, and then stand up. Trust me.

4. Rest, rest, rest! I have no idea what it is like to be pregnant AND have other kids running around. I can only imagine how tough that would be. You ladies deserve a medal...or at least a week long all expenses paid vacation where no one can talk to or touch you. If you are a first-time mom, and even if you aren't, try to rest as much as possible. If I miss anything about my pre-baby life, it is alone time and REST.

Caution

Before moving on I feel the need to warn you about something no one told me about my first trimester...do not eat foods you love because you may end up hating them. Save it for your second trimester when you're feeling better, and your third trimester when you turn into a dinosaur and eat everything in sight. I used to love Subway sandwiches and got them all the time for lunch. The few times I felt good enough to eat something besides crackers, I chose Subway sandwiches. TO THIS DAY I can no longer stand even the smell of Subway. Being pregnant completely killed my love of subs...a tragedy for anyone too lazy to toast their own sandwiches. Something about the smell and taste is now associated with nausea and I just can't do it. Why no one told me that morning sickness may make you hate foods you love, I don't know. But, I love you enough to tell you. Wait until your feel better to eat your favorite foods, just in case.

To Eat or Not to Eat...

Once you start feeling better, you will probably be pretty excited to start eating normal foods again. I feel like there should be a pamphlet at the OB's office next to all the other ones that lists what foods are safe and not safe during pregnancy, since no one told me! I literally had to Google everything before I ate it because I was so paranoid.

Listeria

The biggest thing you need to watch out for is listeria. According to the FDA, listeria monocytogenes is a harmful bacterium that can be found in refrigerated, ready-to-eat foods such as meat, poultry, seafood, and dairy - unpasteurized milk and milk products or foods made with unpasteurized milk It can also be found in produce harvested from soil contaminated with listeria. So, what does this mean for you mama? It means you should AVOID the foods from this list below, courtesy of the FDA:

1. Hot dogs, deli meats, and lunch meats, unless they are cooked until hot.

2. Soft cheeses like Feta, Brie, and Camembert, "blue-veined cheeses," or "queso blanco," "queso fresco," or Panela. Unless these cheeses are made with pasteurized milk, they should be avoided during pregnancy. Always make sure the label says, "made with pasteurized milk".

3. Refrigerated pâtés or meat spreads.

4. Refrigerated smoked seafood, unless it's in a cooked dish, such as a casserole. This includes salmon, trout, whitefish, cod, tuna, and mackerel. These types of seafood are most commonly labeled as "nova-style," "lox," "kippered," "smoked," or "jerky" and can be found in the refrigerator section or sold at deli counters of grocery stores.

5. Raw (unpasteurized) milk or foods that contain unpasteurized milk. As I mentioned before, always read the labels to be sure your dairy products and food are made with pasteurized milk.

Other Foods to Avoid

The foods listed above are considered high risk for contracting listeria and should not be consumed until after the baby is born. Unfortunately, there are more foods and drinks you should avoid during pregnancy even though they aren't a listeria threat. They include:

1. High mercury seafood such as shark, swordfish, bigeye tuna, marlin, king mackerel, and tilefish. According to the FDA, pregnant women can eat up to 12 ounces of low-mercury fish and shellfish a week, but I chose to just avoid them altogether.

2. Fresh-squeezed juice. Pasteurized juice (such as juice from a carton at the grocery store) is considered safe but you should avoid going to juice bars (I know, ugh). The FDA states that when unwashed fruits and vegetables are peeled, cut, or fresh-squeezed, harmful bacteria that may be on the outside can spread to the inside of the produce. You never know if the fruits and veggies you are

consuming are properly cleaned, unless you do it yourself.

3. Sushi. I know, I know, this one about killed me too. Luckily, you CAN eat the vegetarian sushi rolls because they don't contain any meat or fish. You're welcome!

4. Energy drinks and alcohol. Because duh.

5. Unwashed fruits and veggies. Although most fruits are considered safe during pregnancy, you should avoid papaya, grapes (even raisins), and pineapple as they may trigger early labor and can affect your baby. Always wash your fruits and veggies before eating them. I recommend getting a fruit wash from Amazon or your grocery store to be sure they are bacteria free! As always, check the label to see if there are any pesky chemicals hiding in the ingredients before picking a fruit and veggie wash.

6. Don't lick the spoon when baking. Cookie dough, brownie mix, and cake batter made with raw eggs can be really dangerous. I know it sucks, trust me I am an avid spoon licker, but it isn't good for you or your growing babe.

7. Soft-serve ice cream and frozen yogurt. Say what? I know…but those machines at the self-serve ice cream and yogurt places can be a breeding ground for listeria. The employees are required to clean the machines on a regular basis, but you just never know how thoroughly they actually do it. Buy some frozen yogurt from the grocery store instead but be sure the label says it was made with pasteurized milk. Better safe than sorry!

To All My Caffeine Queens

Even though this one isn't on my list, I feel that it is my duty as a coffee lover to let my fellow coffee lovers know that you don't have to completely give up caffeine! *Que the hallelujah chorus* Believe it or not, my doctor actually "prescribed" me a cup of coffee a day to combat my migraines. Obviously, don't go overboard, avoid added creams and sugar, and always check with your doctor first, but a cup of coffee a day should not hurt your baby.

Poking and Prodding

Before I get into this, please keep in mind that I am not a doctor or a nutritionist, and you can make whatever decisions you feel are best for you during your pregnancy. I am not here to sway you one way or another. My goal is to educate you on the things no one talked to me about, so you can make informed decisions on what you feel is best for you and your baby. Talk to your doctor about any concerns you have, but also listen to your mom intuition. Research everything you feel iffy about, so you can decide for yourself. This is YOUR pregnancy, not anyone else's.

How Often Will You See Your Doctor?

You can expect to see your doctor about once a month during weeks 4-28, every other week during weeks 28-36, and every week from week 36 until birth. This can vary if you are high risk, but typically this is how often your doctor will want to see you. It is very common for your doctor to take a urine sample every time you visit them. The reason for this, according to Americanpregnancy.org, is to assess bladder or kidney infections, diabetes, dehydration and preeclampsia by screening for high levels of sugars, proteins, ketones and bacteria. You can also expect to be weighed, have your blood pressure taken, have a visual examination, your belly measured, and the best part...listen to your baby's heartbeat! It is a good idea to write down any questions you have and bring them with you to your appointment, so you can discuss them with your OB.

Your First Visit

During your first visit, you will most likely have your blood drawn, urine tested, receive a pap smear (same as your annual visit) and your first ultrasound! A pap smear is done during your first visit to test for any sexually transmitted diseases and to be sure there aren't any abnormal cells. Rest assured that if anything does come back abnormally, they have pregnancy safe antibiotics and treatments for them. I feel the need to tell you that your first ultrasound will most likely be an internal one, not the one that goes on your belly. I was quite shocked during my first visit to discover they would have to do an internal ultrasound because the baby is so small. It really isn't that bad (although I wish I had done some landscaping first), and you forget all about what's going on the second you see your baby. You may even get to hear the heartbeat! I lovingly referred to my baby as a parasite after seeing her for the first time because she looked like a moth in a cocoon hanging from the side of my uterus.

Heart Beats and Rates

You may not be able to physically see your baby during every visit, but you should be able to hear the heart beat! They say that your baby is more likely to be a boy if the heart rate is below 140 beats per minute and a girl if it is over 140 bpm. My daughter's heart rate was consistently 152-160 bpm, so I had a suspicion she was a she! You won't find out the gender until between weeks 16-20, but it is fun to guess based off old wives' tales and the beats per minute.

Genetic Testing

During your second trimester you may be offered genetic testing. These tests range in invasiveness and are done for many different purposes. If you have a family history of certain genetic disorders, or if you are concerned about Down Syndrome, you may want to consider them. I personally turned down any additional genetic testing, but you can do some research if your doctor suggests it before deciding.

Group B Strep

During your third trimester, it is recommended that you get tested for Group B Strep. According to What to Expect.com, Group B strep (GBS) is a type of common bacteria normally found in the vaginas of many healthy women (estimates are between 10 and 35 percent of all women). It is harmless to those who have it, but without treatment it can be transmitted to the baby during childbirth. This can lead to an infection, so it is recommended you have the test done to rule it out. The test is performed similarly to a pap smear, and the results will be sent to a lab for analysis. If you do have it, don't worry, you will most likely be given antibiotics that are safe to take while pregnant and everything should be fine!

Vaccines

There are also 2 vaccines that are recommended during your third trimester. Please remember that you can accept or deny these vaccines so never let your doctor pressure you into doing them if you are against it. The first one is the flu shot, typically recommended to women who are pregnant during flu season (November-March). I personally turned down this vaccine because I don't get flu shots regularly. I decided to continue to eat healthy, avoid crowded places, and wash my hands a lot. But I know plenty of women who did choose to receive it and are totally fine with healthy babies. The second one is the Tdap (Tetanus toxoid, reduced diphtheria toxoid and acellular pertussis). I did choose to have this vaccine because it protects your baby from whooping cough (pertussis) once they are born. Both the flu and pertussis can be extremely dangerous for newborns, so it is a good idea to have your partner or anyone planning on being around the baby to receive one or both vaccines as well.

P.S.

Lamaze and child birthing classes may terrify you. I chose to avoid these classes like the plague and just did my own research instead. That way, when I felt like I was going to throw up, I could just put on a movie instead of pretending like everything was fine in front of an entire class of pregnant women. Some women would probably disagree with me, but I didn't take a single class and never wanted to. Why pay the money when you have Google and YouTube? To each her own but I would much rather have a panic attack in the comfort of my own home.

Anatomy Scan and Gender Reveal

Now back to the fun stuff! If you want to know the gender ahead of time, it is literal torture to have to wait 16-20 weeks to find out. I counted down for months. During this appointment, they will do what's called an anatomy ultrasound, so it takes a little longer than your regular appointments. The anatomy ultrasound includes measurements of your baby, as well as checking the brain, face, heart, spine, and major organs for any abnormalities. They will also check your anatomy to be sure your placenta is positioned correctly and see if there is enough amniotic fluid for your baby to move around in. And of course, you should be able to find out the gender! Although the ultrasound technician is not allowed to say they are 100% certain it is a boy or a girl, it's very rare that they are wrong. When mine told me I was having a girl I was so excited and kept trying to get her to promise me my baby wouldn't somehow morph into a boy. She told me she wasn't allowed to say she is 100% sure, but she did say that my baby "definitely did not have a penis". That was good enough for me!

Gender Reveal Parties

If you've never heard of a gender reveal party, hop on Pinterest and check out all the fun ways you can tell your family and friends if you're having a boy or a girl. Or, you could even have them be the ones who surprise you! The ultrasound tech can write the gender down on a piece of paper and put it in an envelope, so you can't see it. Then, you can take that envelope and give it to a family member to plan the reveal, or even a bakery to make a cake with pink or blue frosting inside. There are tons of ways to find out the gender of your baby whether you are doing the surprising or you are the one being surprised. For me, I couldn't wait a second longer, so I needed to know as soon as possible. We had some friends and family over later that day and we ordered pizzas. I wrote "It's A..." in one box, and "GIRL!" in the other. That way, when everyone gathered around to eat, they were all surprised to see it was a girl. Since not all our family and friends could be there for that reveal, we had a second one the next day. I baked cupcakes and had everyone bite into them at the same time revealing pink frosting inside. I must warn you that even though the cupcake reveal was a blast, cupcake crumbs will fly from the mouths of your loved ones like rain during monsoon season from excitement, so you may want to stand back a reasonable distance.

There are so many fun ways to announce the gender so don't skimp on this part. It will be one of the first memorable moments of your pregnancy journey and you'll look back on it forever. Take a lot of pictures for your scrapbook or just to have so you can show your baby how excited everyone was to meet him/her!

The "I Love Being Pregnant" Trimester

The second trimester is from weeks 13-28, and most women feel great during this time! Unfortunately, there are some women who suffer with sickness and complications during their entire pregnancy, but for the most part this trimester is the best one. I felt so much better, my belly was the perfect size, and I was able to start feeling my baby move around and kick. You can expect to start feeling your baby move between weeks 16-25, and typically women pregnant with their first baby may not feel them until closer to 25. I'm gonna be real with you, at first, it's hard to tell if it is your baby moving or if you're just gassy. But don't worry because you will have plenty of time to feel that baby move, hiccup, and kick you in the ribs. Don't rush it.

My Second Trimester Essentials

I didn't really need much to "survive" this trimester but there are a few items (added onto some from the first trimester essentials) that helped. These items include:

Burt's Bees Mama Bee Belly Butter
A Super Comfy Adjustable Bra
Tums
Healthy Snacks
Maternity Clothes
Notebook and Pens

1. Burt's Bees Mama Bee Belly Butter was what I used to prevent stretch marks, but there are quite a few options out there for this inevitable side effect. I also used pure coconut oil and I am proud to announce I didn't get any stretch marks during my

pregnancy. Woo hoo right? Don't hate me yet. Here's something no one told me about stretch marks…those jerks can show up AFTER you give birth when everything is deflating. Even though I obsessively used my oils and my lotions, I still got stretch marks. But here is another thing no one told me about stretch marks…I love them! I like to think of them as battle scars from growing a tiny person for 40 weeks! Not to mention, almost every mom has them, even celebrities. Not all of us are blessed with perfectly photoshopped pictures post-birth, so don't sweat it. Put your lotion and oil on your chest, hips, belly, and thighs and if you do end up getting them, then rock those tiger stipes honey!

2. Finding a bra that is extra comfortable is extremely important during this trimester. I couldn't believe how big my boobs got and how quickly it happened! I know all of you small breasted girls are getting excited but hang on a sec. I was 5 feet tall, 119 pounds, and was wearing a 36 DD bra during my second trimester. I about had a heart attack when the woman at Dillard's took my measurements. Yes, that's right ladies…Dillard's. Say bye bye to Victoria's Secret because at this point the twins will take over and you'll need support. And they only get bigger as your pregnancy progresses and when your milk comes in (more on that later). Mine were literally resting on my belly by the time I gave birth. Super sexy. But honestly, at that point I would have worn plastic bags from the dollar store if it meant they were contained.

3. A lot of women experience heartburn and indigestion during their pregnancy, so having Tums

nearby can offer some relief. As your baby grows, all your internal organs get smooshed around to make room, so it isn't uncommon to have digestive issues during this time. I carried some with me throughout the day and kept them by my bed at night to help settle my tummy when I needed it.

4. Keeping healthy snacks with you is a good way to avoid giving in to unhealthy cravings when you are out and about. Trust me, I was constantly tempted to grab a cookie while I was out running errands because, well, I was pregnant, and I was allowed! To fight these urges, I kept healthy snacks in my purse and next to my bed in case I got hungry. Try trail mix, dried fruit, protein or granola bars, and whole wheat crackers.

5. I didn't start gaining weight until about halfway through my pregnancy, but maternity clothes definitely came in handy when I did finally "pop". The bottoms have high waisted stretchy bands and most of the tops have scrunchy sides. They are designed to grow with you as your belly gets bigger, so you shouldn't have to buy a bunch of different sizes. Speaking of gaining weight, you can expect to gain up to 40 pounds during your pregnancy depending on your body type. According to WebMD, you should gain about 2-4 pounds during the first three months you're pregnant and 1 pound a week during the rest of your pregnancy. This is different if you are expecting twins. In that case, you should gain 35 to 45 pounds during your pregnancy. This would be an average of 1 ½ pounds per week after the usual weight gain in the first three months. I gained a total of 40 pounds so don't stress about it. I may have felt like a beluga whale,

but my baby and I were healthy! Just try to eat clean and stay active.

6. The final item I recommend keeping with you is a notebook and pen(s). I would be driving and randomly have a question pop into my head for my doctor. As soon as I stopped I would write the question down in my notebook so I wouldn't forget it. Pregnancy brain is no joke! You will forget things all the time and it's a bigger pain than your swollen feet. You can also use your notebook to keep track of your To-Do lists if you're a type A person, like me.

Leaky Boob Syndrome

Before moving on, I feel the need to share with you another little tidbit that no one ever told me could happen during your pregnancy…leaky boob syndrome. Okay, so that's not the actual name for it, but in all seriousness I was leaking clear fluids randomly throughout the day. I learned that it was colostrum, aka liquid gold, aka baby superfood (more on this later). You can start to produce colostrum as early as your first trimester! Don't worry, it isn't enough to soak through a bra or anything, but it did freak me out at first. I started producing it during my third trimester and learned it wasn't a big deal. Thank you, Google, because there was no way I was going to ask anyone about this. Also, your nipples will be the size of a small country. Sorry.

The Gross Juice Test

You may or may not know that you can develop a certain type of diabetes while pregnant. It's called gestational diabetes, and I had never heard about it before. I learned from my doctor that I would need to undergo a blood test to see if I had it or not between weeks 24-28 of my pregnancy. It is important to know if you have gestational diabetes because if it is left undetected, it can lead to high blood pressure, preeclampsia, preterm labor, and a difficult birth leading to a C section. The risk factors for your baby include high birth weight, heart disease, respiratory distress, and more.

Who is at Risk?

Gestational diabetes is not necessarily based off your weight. Even women who gain little weight during their pregnancy can develop it. It all depends on how pregnancy affects your body's ability to process glucose and if it causes higher than normal blood sugar levels. Anyone can develop gestational diabetes during pregnancy, even though it is relatively rare. However, according to Everydayhealth.com, you are more at risk if you are overweight, have high blood pressure, are prediabetic, had gestational diabetes with a previous pregnancy, have a family history of type 2 diabetes, are of a certain ethnicity, or are over the age of 25. Eating a healthy diet and exercising will lower your risk of developing it.

What Happens During the Test?

First, you will take home a type of juice that contains glucose. It is a very sugary tasting drink called Glucola, usually in an orange or fruit punch flavor. Some women I've talked to said they were told not to eat anything that morning, and to drink the juice on an empty stomach before having their blood drawn. A lot of these women ended up feeling very ill, and some even threw up from it. I brought these concerns to my doctor, and she told me I could eat some bland food that morning such as egg whites or toast to go with the juice. Check with your doctor, but there should not be any reason you have to drink it on an empty stomach. There is a time limit on how quickly you must finish the juice, but your doctor will go over all of this with you, so don't worry.

After eating a bland breakfast and drinking my juice, I headed to my doctor to have my blood drawn. Typically, you will need to have your blood drawn within the hour. My blood test came back normal, meaning I did not develop gestational diabetes.

What Happens if You Have Elevated Levels?

If yours does come back with elevated levels, you will have to go back and do a 3-hour glucose tolerance test. For this test, you cannot eat or drink anything (besides sips of water) for 8-14 hours before. You will have your blood tested before drinking the juice, and then three times every hour after drinking the juice. If you do end up having gestational diabetes, don't panic! Through a healthy diet, exercise, and sometimes taking medication, you can get it under control. The good news is, your blood sugar should return to normal soon after you give birth! You will still need to work with your doctor because there is a risk for developing type 2 diabetes, but most women return to normal after delivery.

Glucola and Your Health

Having said all of that, I do feel inclined to let you know (because I love you) that the Glucola drink is not the best thing for your health. I didn't find out about this until after I took the test and began researching it, but I wish that I had. I assumed that because my doctor told me I needed to do it, then it was safe. To be clear, I had no side effects from the drink and my baby is completely healthy. I also don't personally know any women who had side effects (aside from the drink making them feel icky). But, knowing what I know now, I probably would have decided against the juice and done the test a different way. Here is the ingredient list for the orange flavor Glucola drink. Feel free to look up more details on the risks associated with them:

- Water
- Dextrose: Made from corn syrup and can lead to your child having allergies to corn. Also, a lot of corn syrup is derived from GMO corn.
- Citric Acid: Though found naturally in citrus fruits, the type of citric acid found in our everyday foods is made through industrial production. Definitely not the same.
- Natural Flavoring: Do not be fooled when anything is labeled as "natural". The FDA does not require companies to elaborate on what exactly the natural flavoring is, but it was most likely created in a lab, though derived from natural sources.
- Modified Food Starch: A close cousin to MSG

- Glycerol Ester of Wood Rosin: An oil-soluble food additive found in many sports drinks, cosmetics, and chewing gum.
- Brominated Soybean Oil: Also approved as a flame retardant.
- Artificial Food Dyes: If you ever see anything with artificial food dies in them, run! Red #40, Blue #1, Yellow #6, etc. are all examples of these dangerous chemicals that can lead to cancer. The orange flavor Glucola contains FD&C Yellow #6. FD&C is a synthetic dye used in foods, drugs, and cosmetics.
- Sodium Hexametaphosphate: An additive used to prevent mineral corrosion. Also used in bubble bath, pet food, and teeth whitening products.
- BHA: A proven carcinogen also used to keep food from going bad.
- Sodium Benzoate: A common food preservative especially dangerous when found in canned food and drinks.

What Are Some Alternatives?

According to the Centers for Disease Control and Prevention, only 2-10% of pregnant women develop gestational diabetes. But, as I mentioned before, it is important to know if you have it or not. There are symptoms to watch out for, such as excessive thirst, frequent urination, excessive fatigue, etc. Because these symptoms are also common pregnancy symptoms in general, it is important to rule it out. Here are some alternatives to the Glucola Test:

1. You could turn down the test altogether. I don't recommend this because of the risks involved, but you do have the right to turn down any tests you are

not comfortable with. Discuss concerns with your doctor, but ultimately this is not a test you have to do.

2. The Jelly Bean Test. This is exactly what it sounds like and quite frankly, I totally would have jumped on board with this one, had I known it was an option. Though it is said to be not as accurate as the Glucola, the jelly bean test has you eat 28 jelly beans (totaling 50 grams of sugar) and then test your blood sugar. There are jelly beans out there that are organic and don't contain any scary ingredients. Check out Surf Sweets Organic Jelly Beans by Wholesome. They are made with all-natural sweeteners, no artificial colors or flavors, they're vegetarian, and non-GMO. You can purchase them online from the Natural Candy Store. Be sure that they total 50 grams of sugar though!

3. Random Blood Testing. You can actually buy your own glucose testing kit on Amazon! They range in price from about $30-$60 and you can test your levels randomly throughout your pregnancy to be sure you aren't developing gestational diabetes.

The "Everything Hurts and I'm Dying" Trimester

The third trimester can be a really busy time for expecting moms. You're most likely planning your baby shower, organizing all the baby stuff, and nesting like crazy. I'm here to tell you that nesting is absolutely a real thing. I was painting my entire house, cleaning all the tile grout, and vacuuming the tops of my ceiling fans like a woman who had just been told Oprah was on her way over. As soon as I finished one project, I found another. I had this irresistible urge to make everything as perfect as possible before my baby arrived. As fun as nesting is, you should also take it easy during this time too, as your ligaments are under a lot of stress and you can hurt yourself easily.

My Third Trimester Essentials

Here are a few essential items I found and used religiously to get me though the final trimester:

A Maternity Belly Band
Exercise/Birth Ball
Dry Shampoo
Slippers
Foot and Leg Lotion
Netflix

1. Buying a belly band was one of the smartest things I could have done for myself during those last few months. When you're carrying around a baby that's about to fall out, a belly band offers some much-needed support. There are a ton of options on Amazon to choose from, but I picked a simple pink

one that was adjustable. They wrap around your waist and help hold your belly up a little, relieving all that pressure. I wore mine almost constantly on top of my clothes. They're affordable too, so grab one and I promise you'll thank me for it.

2. I purchased my exercise/birthing ball at Target for about $10 and bounced on it all the time during my third trimester. Not only does bouncing on the ball increase blood flow to your baby and oxygen to its house (your uterus) like a houseplant, but it also relieves spinal pressure and helps with aching legs, knees, and ankles. If you're about to give birth, a birthing ball can also help move the baby down and into the correct position for birth. I had an emergency C section so that benefit didn't apply to me, but I do know a few women who it helped tremendously! If anything, it's super fun so just do yourself a favor and get one.

3. Can we all just take a moment and thank the good Lord above for whoever invented dry shampoo? I mean seriously, what a magical invention that allows us to go days without having to wash our hair and not look homeless! Dry shampoo will become your new best friend once you have the baby, so you might as well stock up now! I was lucky enough to give birth in January when it's cool outside but if you are super pregnant during the summer months, washing and blow drying your hair may sound like literal torture. On the days I was too tired to do my hair, dry shampoo came to my rescue. I also had to be very careful after my C section about taking showers so dry shampoo was my hero. It will help dry up any oil on your hair from not washing it. My favorite brand is the

Kristin Ess one from Target because it smells AMAZING and helped mask the smell of spit up that was all over me when my daughter was nursing.

4. Slippers are heavenly on swollen feet when your baby is almost here. I was due during the wintertime, so my feet were always cold. Your feet may also grow while you're pregnant so getting some soft, cozy slippers will help with any aching.

5. Speaking of aching feet, investing in some therapeutic foot and leg lotion during the last few weeks of pregnancy can be magical. Find one with peppermint in it to relieve sore muscles and give your legs and feet a good rub down. You could also go get a pedicure and bring the lotion with you for the nail technician to use! Your body tends to swell a little right before you give birth and your muscles will be sore. Burt's Bees Mama Bee Leg and Foot Cream is a great natural brand, and it smells awesome.

6. Netflix was a Godsend during those last few weeks when I had trouble sleeping. I loved to be out on the couch with my Snoogle and binge watch Netflix. Everyone told me to enjoy the last few weeks and days before the baby came and boy were they right! I miss those nights where I could just sit on the couch alone, eat whatever I wanted, and watch every TV show Netflix offered. You may be extremely uncomfortable and need to pee every 5 minutes, but seriously try to enjoy this time alone. As great as being a mom is, I do miss my alone time.

Red Raspberry Leaf Tea

Before moving on I wanted to talk about red raspberry leaf tea, which is something you may or may not have heard of. If you have a midwife or a doula, then you probably have heard of it, but if not, I want to inform you about the possible risks and benefits of drinking it during your pregnancy. Red raspberry leaf tea is exactly what it sounds like...tea made from the leaves of the red raspberry plant. It is NOT the same as red raspberry tea, which is usually just raspberry flavored black tea.

There is still a lot of debate on whether the tea works or not, and some women feel very strongly one way or the other. It is said to have been used for centuries for womb wellness and uterus toning, which promotes a faster and easier pregnancy, with less chance of medical intervention. According to thebump.com, "it provides B vitamins, iron, niacin, manganese, magnesium, selenium, vitamin A and astringent alkaloids that nourish and contribute to the healing process," says Eden Fromberg, MD, board-certified ob-gyn and medical director at Holistic Gynecology in New York City. It is recommended that you start drinking a cup of the tea once a day around 32 weeks, and gradually increase your intake as your due date approaches. Some women believe that the tea works as a softening agent, which helps prepare the cervix and uterus for labor.

Thebump.com also states that even though the American Pregnancy Association says that red raspberry leaf tea is "likely safe" during pregnancy, you should sip with caution since tea manufacturers don't have to get Food and Drug Administration approval. Side effects of drinking the tea may include nausea, diarrhea, an increase in Braxton Hicks contractions, and can also mess with your insulin levels. If you are diagnosed with gestational diabetes, you should not drink red raspberry leaf tea.

A lot of women believe that if they drink the tea around the time they are due, then it will help induce labor. I was one of them. After doing a lot of research, I decided to give it a try. I only did one or two cups of the tea a day for about a week, but I did not notice a difference in anything. My daughter still ended up coming five days past her due date and I had a rough labor, so for me it didn't work. If this is something you are considering trying, be sure to talk to your doctor first and do some research of your own to be sure it is safe for you.

Cha-Ching!

The Baby Registry Wish List

I'm a planner and cannot function without to-do lists so naturally, I did this during my pregnancy as well. I made a list for almost everything and rechecked them about 100 times, just to be sure I covered everything. Lucky for you, I did all this for you too! Keep in mind, you may register for items you don't end up using, and you may not register for items that you end up needing. I put together a list of ALL the items I can think of, so feel free to read about why each one is important and pick and choose which ones you think you'll need. Baby registries are a chance to treat yo' self and get spoiled a little so don't be afraid to pick things you want! Also, you can buy any of these items for yourself too. I certainly picked out a lot of my own stuff that wasn't on my registry.

Furniture

Furniture is not typically something people purchase off registries because it is more expensive and hard to wrap in cute wrapping paper. You would be better off buying furniture yourself or asking for gift cards, so you can pick the specific pieces you want. The furniture you will most likely need include:

1. A Crib and Crib Mattress. A crib is probably the first piece of furniture you think of when planning for a baby, right? Whether you plan to co-sleep or crib train, it is a good idea to purchase or register for a crib, so you have it just in case. Look for a convertible one, so it can grow with your baby and

stay with them through their toddler years if you want to save some money! You will also need a crib mattress that not only fits but is safe too. I recommend reading as many reviews as you can before selecting a specific brand so you can see what other moms loved or didn't love about the crib and mattress you want.

2. Crib Sheets and Waterproof Mattress Cover. Even if you purchase your crib and mattress yourself, you can still register for a couple adorable fitted sheets. Add at least two waterproof mattress covers too, since babies tend to be messy. It's much easier in the middle of the night to strip the bedding and replace it, than to try and clean stains off the actual mattress. Also, until your baby is older, you should avoid buying comforters and pillows because they can be a suffocation hazard.

3. Comfy Rocking Chair. I know in the old days moms rocked their babies in wooden chairs, and there's nothing wrong with that! But, if you plan to breastfeed I do recommend investing in a comfy rocking chair with a foot rest since you will be spending a lot of time (and quick power naps) there. My daughter is almost three years old and we still like to rock in her chair while I read to her.

4. Changing Table and Changing Pad. I didn't register for a changing table, but I did register for a changing pad and cute covers for it. I went to Goodwill and found a changing table for about $15, painted it white, and added adorable knobs from Hobby Lobby so it matched the nursery. If you do register for a changing table, they can be a little pricey so you may be better off using gift cards or

buying one yourself. Changing pads are in between the most and least purchased baby registry items so they are worth adding. Pick several covers for them that will coordinate with your nursery theme as well.

5. Dresser or Clothing Storage Unit. I don't know a single mama who registered for a dresser and actually got it. Unless it was from their parents or a relative who wanted to buy all the furniture. As with the other large items, you can save your gift cards or purchase them yourself. I am a huge fan of Goodwill shopping and redoing pieces of furniture myself, but if that isn't your style, check out Ikea. I used one of those cube storage systems with matching baskets to store baby socks, pants, etc. and it worked perfectly!

6. Bookshelf. People LOVE to get books for babies, and some moms even ask that people bring books with notes written in them instead of cards (how cute!). You will need a place to store all these books, so it is safe to register for a little bookshelf if you want. It doesn't need to be a big one, and it's good to have it low to the floor for safety reasons.

Baby Gear Necessities

Now that we've gone over the basics for the nursery furniture, let's get into the gear your baby will need specifically. These are still relatively large items, but you have a good chance of receiving them off your registry because babies use them a bunch!

1. High Chair. Your baby won't be able to sit in a high chair for a while, but it is a great item to register for so you have it in the future. I kept mine in the box until my daughter was big enough for it.

2. Pack 'n Play. Pack 'n Plays are awesome for a lot of reasons. My grandmother got me one with a changing table and a bassinet for when my daughter was a newborn, but there are a few options based on your needs. As your baby gets older, they can play in them safely while you get some house chores done! I brought my Pack 'n Play to work with me, so my daughter could play and nap while I got stuff done. It was nice because I didn't have to worry about her crawling all over the floor. Also, my niece slept in hers next to my brother's bed for two years, so they are very versatile.

3. Co-Sleeper. If you plan to breastfeed, investing in a co-sleeper will save your sanity. Depending on how you want to sleep train, co-sleepers allow your baby to safely sleep next to you, rather than in another room in their crib. Your newborn will want to eat every few hours and it may be hard to go all the way into another room when you are exhausted. I ended up co-sleeping with my daughter and never used my actual crib, but I did try out a few different co-sleepers before I felt comfortable. Having your

baby in bed with you can be dangerous, so find a co-sleeper you feel would be best for you. Some of the top brands include the SwaddleMe By Your Side Sleeper, the DockaTot, the Snuggle Nest Harmony, and the Halo Bassinet Glide Sleeper.

4. Baby Swing. Baby swings are perfect for when you need a break from holding your baby and need to get some work done around the house. Most play music and have mobiles so your baby will be infatuated with it. They also rock themselves which keep babies very happy when they aren't in their mama's arms.

5. Baby Rocker. This is different from the baby swing because they are more portable and don't need an outlet. I absolutely LOVED the Fisher-Price Rock n Play Sleeper. I used it for my daughter's naps, while I cooked, while I showered, etc. My sister-in-law let me borrow hers, but they are a great item to register for.

6. Baby Play Mat and Activity Center. These are so much fun, especially when you start doing tummy time with your baby. I received the Skip Hop brand at my baby shower and my daughter loved it. Activity mats usually come with mirrors, hanging toys, music, and even a C shaped pillow to put under the chest to encourage neck strengthening. This was one of the first items purchased off my registry so find your favorite and add it!

Travel Items

Again, any of these items can be registered for or bought yourself based off the specific brands you like. I found a lot of items on Amazon but didn't have an Amazon registry, so I bought them myself. I'm also picky...don't judge me. Here are the most important travel items your baby will need:

1. Infant Car Seat. A car seat is one of the top most important items your baby will need in general. The hospital won't let you leave without one and will even help you get it adjusted perfectly so you know your baby is safe. I highly recommend starting with an actual infant car seat rather than one that converts to a toddler car seat. Convertible car seats are made to stay put in the car. Infant car seats allow you to pop them in and out of the car and carry them with you. If you are worried about expense, some stores offer trade in events where you can bring your old car seat to the store and get a discount on a new one. You'll need a convertible car seat once your baby outgrows the infant one, but you typically have at least a year before that happens. You can also sell your used infant car seat but beware. Check the expiration date and be sure it is in perfect condition, so the next baby is safe too! I registered for a car seat/stroller combo, so I knew for sure that car seat would fit in it.

2. Stroller. As I mentioned above, I found a car seat and stroller combo that matched but if you get them separately don't worry! Just be sure your stroller can accommodate an infant car seat. Trust me, it is heaven when you can pop that heavy car seat into a stroller and go. Also find one with good reviews

that is lightweight and easily collapsible. You will be juggling a lot of stuff when you're out with your baby so having a lightweight stroller will help you a bunch.

3. Car Mirror. I was such a freak after my daughter was born thanks to postpartum anxiety that I relied heavily on my car mirror to see her in the back seat. Because she was rear facing, I was unable to see her without it. Obviously, it is not safe to turn your whole body around while driving, so register for a car mirror that attaches to the head rest above your baby. You will be able to glance in your rearview mirror and see your bundle of love without putting yourself in danger.

4. Sunshades. I registered for sunshades to protect my baby from the sun. We live in Arizona, so the sun here is brutal. Sunshades attach to the windows in the back, so you never have to worry if your baby is getting burned.

5. Backseat Organizer. You may not actually use this until your baby is a little older, but they still come in handy. Backseat organizers attach to the back of the driver or passenger side seats and can hold wipes, diapers, a change of clothes, water bottles, a first aid kit, toys, and more. You'll never have to worry about forgetting or needing something while you're out!

6. Car Seat Monitor. These didn't exist when I had my daughter, but they are one of the best inventions, in my opinion, for modern mamas. These monitors clip onto your baby's car seat strap and alert you if the strap comes loose, or if you forget to buckle

them in. I was so tired once that I forgot to buckle my baby in when she was a few weeks old. I know you're thinking that would never happen to you...trust me I thought so too. I was horrified and cried for hours while hugging her. It never would have happened if I had the monitor. An alarm also goes off if you get more than 15 feet away from your baby, so you'll never accidentally leave them anywhere. I know it sounds crazy, but you can read about how many moms accidentally leave their babies in shopping carts or cars. I'm sure that will never happen to you, but this monitor makes sure of it!

7. Baby Carrier. When you're out and about with your baby, they will most likely want to be carried whether they're sleeping or not. Even the smallest baby can lead to tired arms so registering for a baby carrier will take the pressure off your arms and back. You may have to try a few before finding one that works for you, but I found the wrap version worked wonders when my daughter was a newborn. The buckle version worked best when she got older. As your baby grows, they will begin to slouch in the wrap carriers which isn't safe or comfortable. They are great for when they are tiny though because it makes them feel like they are in the womb again. When they become more active and want to explore the world around them, getting one that buckles to your chest is the way to go.

8. Diaper Bag. You should register for a diaper bag, so you can have it fully stocked and ready for when the baby comes. You can even register for more than one so if you do get them all, you can test them out and decide which one you like best and return the

others. I was super picky about my diaper bag. I tried out a normal diaper bag but quickly changed to a backpack one. I liked to carry my baby a lot so the backpack one was much easier than one I had to try and keep on my shoulder. This, of course, is personal preference and there are a bunch of beautiful ones to choose from.

Breastfeeding Necessities and Accessories

I bet you had no idea how much would go into simply feeding your baby, but trust me, you will use all of these at some point. Some moms choose not to register for these items because they can be a little personal. But, if you do choose to register for them I am sure that any mother who has ever breastfed a baby will be glad to hook you up.

1. Breast Pump…Or not. I chose not to register for a pump because I discovered my insurance covered it for me! Check with your provider because you might find that they will pay for it. If not, there are plenty of options out there. I ended up with the Medela Automatic Breast Pump and I loved it. Manual pumps never worked for me, so I don't personally recommend them. Reading reviews online will be the best way to know which pumps are the best.

2. Nursing Pillow. This is one of the first gifts people choose off a registry. The Boppy Nursing Pillow is the most popular, and you can use it for more than just nursing. You can use it during tummy time to prop your baby up, and it even helps your baby learn how to sit up on their own. Register for a few

cute pillow cases to go with it since you will need to wash it frequently.

3. Nursing Tanks and Bras. These can be hard to register for because your chest size will change a lot while you adjust to breastfeeding. You may need to try them on to find which ones are most comfortable and which ones you like best. I always purchased black bras and tank tops because they don't stain or show the actual amount of spit up on you at any given time.

4. Nursing Privacy Cover. I tested out the version that also acts as a baby carrier, car seat cover, scarf, and nursing cover but it didn't work for me. It was way too long, and I was constantly fighting with it. I ended up purchasing a simple one that went over my neck and covered me completely. You will need one when your baby starts screaming in the middle of a store because they're hungry. I promise…this will happen.

5. Nursing Pads. Disposable nursing pads worked best for me because I soaked through them a few times a day (I was a dairy cow). Lansinoh Nursing Pads were my favorite, but you could also try out the reusable ones that are washable.

6. Nipple Cream (haha) But seriously. Your boobs are going to be sore when you first start breastfeeding. Try to find cream with natural ingredients because even if you rinse off before you nurse, your baby could still ingest some of it. I recommend the Organic Nipple Balm by the Honest Company or pure coconut oil.

7. Ice Packs. Ice packs are magical for those first few weeks of breastfeeding. I used Lansinoh TheraPearl 3-in-1 Breast Therapy Pack, which could be used hot or cold. The heat helps for those pesky clogged ducts and the cold helps with soreness.

8. Breastmilk Storage Bags. Self-explanatory. Stock up because if you're like me, you'll be overproducing until your boobs calm down. I got the Medela ones to go with my pump. Sticking with the same brand can ensure they fit properly and prevent leaks and spills. I know they say not to cry over spilled milk, but when that milk is breastmilk…you will cry.

9. Burp Cloths. Lots and lots of burp cloths. You'll go through about 5 of these a day.

10. Milkscreen Strips. These test the amount of alcohol in your breastmilk, so you know if you need to pump and dump or if it's safe to nurse after a night out. Hey, moms need to let loose once in a while! This is a judgement free zone.

11. Bottles. Even if you plan to breastfeed, registering for bottles is a good idea. Around a year old, my daughter started taking bottles of breastmilk along with nursing. I always recommend using glass over plastic for anything and everything, but since glass can be pricier than plastic, registering for them could be a money saver. If you do decide to go the plastic bottle route, be sure to check that they are BPA free and can attach to your breast pump. I loved the Dr. Brown's brand.

12. Bottle Drying Rack. This comes in handy for mom's (like me) who chose to hand wash all the baby bottles. Most bottles these days are dishwasher safe, but if you decide to hand wash, a drying rack is a life saver.

13. Bottle Warmer. Highly recommend. Microwaves can leave hot and cold spots in the milk, but bottle warmers thoroughly heat the milk to the right temperature. This is such a time saver and works for formula babies too!

14. Bottle Brushes for hand cleaning bottles. Get or register for a couple of these because they get gross fast. They even have some now that you can add soap to and with a push of a button, you can clean your bottles super easy.

15. Bottle Sterilizer. To be honest, I didn't even know this existed when I had my daughter. This little gadget sanitizes your bottles for you so you never have to worry about germs.

16. Pacifiers. Your baby may or may not take a pacifier, and some professionals may even try to scare you away from using them. None of it is true. If your baby likes a pacifier, let them have it! I don't know anyone whose baby had nipple confusion or trouble nursing because of a pacifier. I also don't believe babies should be left to self soothe and pacifiers will help you tremendously unless you want to be used as a human one. Register for a few different brands to see which one your baby likes best since they come in all styles and shapes.

Bath Time and Grooming

I know our grandmothers use to bathe us in the kitchen sink, but we now have the option to bathe our babies in actual tubs made just for them. Not to mention all the accessories to go with it. These are all the items you can register for, so your baby will have everything they need to be squeaky clean:

1. Baby Tub. These tubs come in a variety of colors, shapes, and sizes. You can place it in your actual tub or on the counter to bathe your nugget. Most even have a hammock for newborns or some type of padding to keep them comfy.

2. Baby Wash and Shampoo. If you haven't figured this out by now, I am a lover of natural products. I want you to be aware that even though a brand may claim they are made for babies, that does NOT mean they are safe. Some of the biggest baby brands are made with toxic chemicals and skin irritants. Your baby doesn't need to smell like bubblegum...stick to scent free products until you know for sure if your baby has any allergies. Register for brands such as California Baby, Earth Mama Angel Baby, the Honest Company, or my favorite...Shea Moisture.

3. Hooded Towels. Hooded towels are better than regular towels because they keep your baby warmer. Not to mention, they come in unicorn, dinosaur, shark, or pig characters so to say they are a necessity would be an understatement.

4. Wash Cloths. You will go through a lot of these and most come in packages of 6-12. Register for a few sets so when they wear out, you'll have more.

5. Baby First Aid and Grooming Kit. These kits come with nail clippers, combs, brushes, a nose sucker, etc. Basically everything you need!

6. Thermometer. Some of the grooming kits do come with a thermometer, but they can be unreliable. It's best to register for an ear thermometer or a forehead thermometer to go with it so you can take your baby's temperature more accurately and easily.

I want to reiterate the importance of what you put on your baby's skin and staying away from artificial fragrances and anything you can't pronounce. Thinking about these chemicals being absorbed into my daughter's skin was a giant nope. Choose brands that contain all natural and organic ingredients to prevent any skin irritation or allergic reactions.

Potty Needs

Babies go potty A LOT. These are the items you should register for to be sure you are prepared for the massive amount of pee and poo headed your way:

1. Diapers. Diapers. Diapers. Register for newborn, size 1, and size 2. Something no one told me about babies…they come in all shapes and sizes and can outgrow newborn diapers fast. Having a few different sizes comes in handy when your baby outgrows one size overnight (I'm serious this happens). Try to find companies that don't use

chlorine, latex, dyes, or fragrances, which unfortunately most of the popular brands do. I also noticed that a lot of the more popular brands had a very strong chemical smell to them the second I opened the box. The Target brand (Up & Up) didn't! Another issue I ran into with the bigger name brands is that the Velcro on the diaper strap cut up my daughter's legs like a cheese grater. No thank you.

2. Diaper Cream/Rash Cream. Every baby is different, but I used coconut oil for almost every rash my daughter got. I don't recommend the heavy creams or ointments for diaper rash because they can clog the pores and make the rash worse. I also used (and still use) Earth Mama Organic Diaper Balm and it works wonders. Again, be sure to check for all-natural ingredients and go for organic when you can.

3. Baby Wipes. Trust me, you're going to go through these faster than you can imagine. Stock up. Beware of the scented wipes, as they can cause irritation to newborn's sensitive skin. Babyganics Face, Hand, and Baby Wipes, Fragrance Free are my favorite.

4. Diaper Genie and Refill Liners. Some moms never had a diaper genie and didn't miss it. But, I did get one and found it to be very beneficial. As I mentioned, I had a C section so I wasn't able to walk well. Being able to toss the diapers into the Diaper Genie helped me a ton! When my daughter got older, I stopped throwing poops in there because it smelled to high heaven. But, it's convenient to throw pee diapers away so you don't have to walk to the dumpster 100 times a day. The refill liners are

a bit pricey so throw those babies on your registry as well.

5. Wipe Warmer. I live in Arizona, so I never used a wipe warmer. If you have your baby during the wintertime, and you live in a cold part of the world, it may be worth the investment. Otherwise, I found that holding the wipe in my hand for a few seconds warmed it right up. This one is totally up to you!

Bedtime

Next up is all the stuff your baby will need for a good night's sleep. Newborns sleep all the time for the first few weeks, but as they get older it's important to establish a nap and bedtime routine. These are all the items you will need to pull it off:

1. Baby Monitor. Baby monitors are also one of the most purchased items off a registry. I highly recommend a baby monitor with a camera that you can watch from your laptop. I know, I know, our parents and grandparents survived raising us without baby monitors in general, let alone ones with a camera. But, they aren't that much more expensive, and being able to see my baby gave my post-partum anxiety ridden self some much needed peace of mind.

2. Sound Machine. When your baby is a newborn, they can pretty much sleep through a herd of elephants stampeding through your living room. It is a common misconception that if you train your baby to sleep through noise, they will continue to do so through toddlerhood. NOT TRUE. Having a

sound machine helps drown out noise and is incredibly soothing. My daughter is almost 3, and I am still using her sound machine for naps and bedtime. Most play different sounds or music and work as a nightlight.

3. Receiving Blankets. Also known as swaddling blankets, these are very light weight, breathable, and will save your sanity when your baby is screaming at 2am. Newborns only know life in the womb so being exposed to the big scary world may lead to a lot of crying. Wrapping your baby in a swaddle helps them feel safe, secure, and instantly calms them. They have a ton of adorable ones so don't be afraid to register for all the ones you like!

4. Blankets. For the love of all that is holy do not register for blankets. Every grandma within a 500-mile radius will want to knit or sew a blanket for your baby. I received more blankets than I knew what to do with even though I did not register for any. Unless there is a particular one you just cannot live without, rest assured you will receive plenty of blankets. Also, no baby should sleep with a blanket until they are much older, so you will most likely end up storing them until them.

Clothes and Accessories

Clothing and accessories are items you don't need to register for, but still can if you want to. I chose not to register for any clothing, socks, shoes, jammies, etc. but still ended up receiving plenty. I wanted to pick all of the clothes for my daughter and hit up all the second-hand thrift stores I could find! Surprisingly, I found most of her clothes from these stores in perfect condition because babies tend to outgrow clothing fast. Here is the list of items to add to your registry, if you choose to do so:

1. Onesies. Little secret...don't rely only on newborn onesies. You will need to get newborn, 3 month, and 3-6 month onesies because your baby will literally outgrow some sizes overnight. Also, every brand fits differently so a 3 month in one brand may fit like a newborn in another. Get short sleeve and long sleeve onesies so you can dress them accordingly.

2. Socks. Babies feet get cold so having a lot of soft fuzzy socks will keep them nice and cozy.

3. Formal Clothes. Okay, your baby isn't going to the MTV Movie Awards. Chances are they will never wear that formal dress your aunt just had to buy your baby. Instead, you will end up putting your baby in it for a picture and never touching it again. It can be tempting to buy adorable outfits but let me tell you this is the surest way to make your baby super mad. Onesies are the most comfortable so don't invest too much money on expensive outfits. Special occasions are one thing, but for every day you won't need fancy outfits.

4. Shoes. My daughter didn't wear shoes until she was walking. Register for shoes at your own risk. They have a lot of adorable ones, don't get me wrong, but all the shoes my daughter received sat in her closet.

5. Accessories. If you're having a girl, it can be very tempting to register for bows, headbands, and hair clips but I can almost guarantee you will receive plenty of them at your baby shower. I only bought ones that I absolutely loved and to be real with you, she pulled all of them out the second I put them in.

The One Item I Couldn't Live Without

Last but not least…invest in a Snuza Hero Baby Movement Monitor or some other monitor. The Snuza goes for around $100 on Amazon but they are worth EVERY SINGLE PENNY. Having post-partum anxiety after my daughter was born made it very difficult for me to sleep for almost 3 weeks. My girlfriend told me about the Snuza Hero she was using with her twins. This little gadget attaches to your baby's diaper and monitors their breathing. If your baby stops breathing for a few seconds, the device vibrates to stimulate them. If that doesn't work and it doesn't detect stomach movement (breathing in and out) an alarm goes off. I used this while my daughter slept and while she was in the car seat because even with a car mirror, you can't tell if they are breathing while they sleep in the car seat behind you. The peace of mind I got from this device was indescribable. Knowing I could sleep peacefully, and an alarm would wake me if anything happened to my baby made my life so much easier. They also have other options that do the same thing, but the Snuza was my favorite.

Treat Yo' Self

I want to talk about some stuff you can do before the baby comes. This list includes self-care, home care, and preparation ideas so you'll feel at peace and organized when you go into labor.

1. Get your carpets cleaned. Your baby won't be crawling until they are about 6-10 months old on average, but you will probably be sitting on the floor with your baby for tummy time within the first few weeks home. Having your carpets professionally cleaned will clear all that dust and pet hair out of there so your baby won't get covered in gross stuff when they roll around on the floor. Those onesies are precious, don't let dust and hair ruin them! Check Groupon for deals or call around for the best quote.

2. Hire a housekeeper. Even if you can't afford to have a housekeeper come every month (I certainly couldn't) I still had one come while I was in the hospital giving birth, and two weeks after I got home. I actually asked my dad for this as a baby shower gift! It really relieved the stress of trying to keep a clean house while caring for a newborn and recovering from surgery.

3. Wash all your baby clothes. I made sure all my daughter's clothes were washed and ready to go a few weeks before she was due. This takes the stress off when you're juggling a newborn who needs a new onesie every hour (yes, I am serious). My favorite laundry detergent for my daughter was the Seventh Generation Free & Clear one. Seventh

Generation does offer a baby detergent with scents derived from essential oils, but I recommend avoiding ANY scents until your baby is older. Newborns have sensitive skin so going the fragrance-free route is best. Also, your baby may have an allergy to a specific oil or scent. Now that my daughter is older, I love the Method laundry detergent and it smells great! Remember, these clothes will be on your new baby all day long, so invest in safer detergent options for them.

4. Pick a pediatrician. Your baby will visit their pediatrician very soon after they are born for their first check up, so having this done will save you a panic attack when the nurse asks you who their pediatrician is for paperwork. Your baby will most likely be visited by the hospital pediatrician on call after they are born to be examined, but you will still need a separate visit with your personal pediatrician within the week after they come home. Ask your friends, do some research, and even visit some pediatrician offices close by. Ask questions, read reviews, and be sure you are super comfortable with your choice. I went with a doctor recommended by my sister-in-law (she had a great experience with my niece), but I ended up switching to another one pretty quickly. I won't go into detail, but if your pediatrician ever makes you feel like you're an inconvenience for asking questions, say buh-bye!

5. Make freezer meals. So, I didn't end up doing this one, but I wish I had! I had a lot of help my first week home with my daughter between my mom, Will, my grandmother, and visitors. I thought I would be fine once they left, but boy was I wrong! I had a lot of help, up until they had to get back to

their lives and I was left on my own eating frozen pizzas. Freezer meals can be prepared before you have the baby and reheated in the crock-pot or oven for when all the help leaves! Pinterest has a ton of ideas, so create a board, pick your favorites, and stock up!

6. Get your hair and nails done. Once the baby gets here, it will be a while before you can sneak away and get a mani/pedi, let alone find the time to go to the salon to get your roots done. Getting a gel manicure and a fresh haircut and color right before you go into labor will help you feel a little more put together after the baby is born. Go ahead and add in a facial too. You deserve it!

7. Maternity photos. This one should not even be considered as an option, it should be a requirement! You don't have to pay a bunch of money for a professional photographer if that isn't your style, but at least have a friend, your mom, or your partner take some photos of you towards the end of your pregnancy. You will cherish these photos of the last few weeks of that baby being all yours. Around 32 weeks is a perfect since your belly will be super cute, but you won't quite be in the I'm so pregnant I can't breathe phase. I had mine professionally done, but if you choose not to, at least get a cute outfit, find a beautiful location, and take pictures right before sunset. You won't regret it!

8. Schedule a hospital tour. You should set up a time to tour the hospital you are planning to deliver at between weeks 30 and 34 of your pregnancy. This is so important because when you do go into labor, you will know exactly where to go and what to

expect. They will show you where to check in, where you will be examined, a labor and delivery room, and a recovery room.

9. Finish any projects. As I mentioned above, nesting is no joke. Making sure that all the little projects you have going around the house are done in time for the baby will ease so much stress! Use this time to get everything done so you can focus on recovery and bonding once the baby is here. Don't be afraid to hire someone or ask for help. Will asked his friend to come over a few weeks before my daughter was born. I handed them a list of things I needed to get done, and it was SO nice to have help finishing everything.

10. Sleep. Yes, I am going to say this again and again because sleep is something you will miss very much. A lot of us work and have other responsibilities, so enjoy being able to relax, take naps, and sleep in whenever you can.

It's Go Time!

Mama's Hospital Bag

Let's talk hospital bags. No idea where to start? I got you girl. And yes, I said bags…not bag. I had one for me, one for the baby, and one for Will. I had my bags packed and in the car around 38 weeks, but if you are high risk, I suggest putting them in your car around 35 weeks. To start, I will share with you all the items I included in my hospital bag:

1. Folder with all documents. Make Copies of your photo ID, insurance info, social security card, hospital forms and birth plan (if you have one). Check your hospital's website for their forms and ask your doctor ahead of time to be sure you have all the necessary forms filled out before going into labor. My hospital actually let me turn in all my paperwork during our hospital tour, so I didn't have to fill anything out when I went into labor. This was such a relief because no one wants to fill out forms in between contractions. I did keep an extra copy of everything in a folder in my hospital bag though, just in case. Also, include a few copies of your birth plan so you can show it to your nurses and your doctor (more on this later).

2. Healthy snacks. Trail mix, crackers, dried fruit, and basically anything without added sugar. I didn't want to eat during my labor and ended up not eating for almost 27 hours because of the emergency C Section (yikes). Try to munch on healthy snacks when you can to keep up your strength. Also, pack some change for the vending machines in case you crave something.

3. Water bottles. The hospital provides water obviously, but bringing a water bottle from home is good to have in case you need it before you get settled into your delivery room.

4. A pair of soft socks. The hospital does provide non-slip socks for you, but they don't compare to the fluffy soft socks that you can bring with you. It's like heaven on your swollen feet.

5. Soft robe or zip up sweater. These not only help you look less like a hospital patient, but they also make breastfeeding easier. Get a comfortable silk robe or a fluffy new zip up sweater just for the occasion.

6. Lip Balm. Pack at least two. Trust me, you'll be doing a lot of mouth breathing so keeping your lips moisturized will help. Don't pick any with harsh scents as this can lead to nausea.

7. Headbands, hair ties, and a brush. If you're like me and can't shower for a few days after birth, headbands keep the baby hairs out of your face and let's face it, a messy bun is the only look you can rock at that point.

8. At least two nursing bras or tanks (if you plan to breastfeed). Here's something no one told me about breastmilk...it may not come in for a few days! My daughter was cluster feeding constantly so my boobs were out almost the entire time. Nursing bras and tanks offer easy access.

9. Toiletries. Travel sized items are the best, and if you can't find your favorite shampoo/conditioner/body wash in those sizes, the travel section at Target has empty bottles you can squeeze them into. Don't forget:

    a. Shampoo and Conditioner
    b. Body wash
    c. Deodorant
    d. Face Wash/Face Wipes
    e. Body Lotion
    f. Dry Shampoo
    g. Moisturizer

10. Loose fitting clothing. Whether you have a vaginal birth or a C section, you are going to be sore. Pack loose fitting clothing that you can easily get on and off so you'll be comfortable. I felt like I was sweating to death most of the time, so make sure you pack both cool and warm clothes.

11. Magazines or a book. Believe it or not, labor can take forever. It's nice to have as many things to take your mind off it as possible.

12. Blanket. I bought a super soft blanket specifically for my daughter's birth. I am so glad I did because I still use it to snuggle her and have all the memories from when she was born.

13. Perineal Spray. Yes, this is a spray for your hoo-ha. Since I didn't give birth vaginally I never used mine, but if you do have a natural birth, this stuff will help soothe your lady parts and any stitches you may have. Check out the Earth Mama Herbal Perineal Spray which eases the discomfort of

postpartum soreness and swelling, helps with the pain from episiotomies and soothes hemorrhoids.

Last Minute Items:

1. Cell phone and charger
2. Headphones
3. Ipad or tablet and charger. Hospital movies aren't too bad…but they have Wifi so bring your tablet and watch Netflix or your favorite downloaded movies.
4. Eyeglasses, contacts, contact solution.
5. Makeup Bag. Hats off to all you ladies who looked like a supermodel after giving birth because I looked like I had been hit by a bus. I packed makeup but never touched it.
6. Toothpaste and Toothbrush. I bought a separate set to bring to the hospital but if you are bringing it from home, don't forget to grab these before you go!

Optional Items For Mama

1. Towels. The hospital provides plenty of these, but they aren't as comfy as the ones you have at home. They take up a lot of space in your bag but can be comforting to have when you finally get to shower. Also, consider leaving a towel in the car for the trip to the hospital, in case your water breaks on the way there.

2. Pads and Granny Panties. I packed these but never used them. I can't speak for the women who give birth vaginally but for you C section mamas, take advantage of the hospitals pads and disposable

mesh underwear for as long as you can. And ask if you can take some home with you. I'm not sure why you can't buy the mesh underwear in bulk at Costco, but you can't. These treasures are only available at the hospital and they are AMAZING. Snag as many as you can. You may be laughing and thinking you wouldn't be caught dead in mesh undies and I get it! I thought the same thing...but you will change your mind. I won't say I told ya so.

3. Hairdryer/Hair Straightener. Girl if you have time to actually blow dry your hair after giving birth we can't be friends. Just kidding (kinda). If you have a birth or newborn photographer coming to the hospital, or you're just a superhero, then you're allowed.

4. Your Own Pillow. I chose not to bring my pillow from home because I didn't want it to get gross or forget it. The hospital has a billion pillows and you can use as many as you want. But, during labor it may be comforting to have a pillow from home. Just be sure to put it in a colored pillow case so you don't lose it!

5. Nursing Pillow. I packed mine but didn't use it. Like I said, the hospital has SO many pillows I just used theirs to nurse her until I got home. But, it isn't a bad thing to bring yours, so you can have help while getting used to it.

6. Vitamins and Medicine. If your doctor prescribed you medication, then obviously bring it. But you don't have to pack things like Tylenol since the hospital can provide everything you need for pain management.

7. Camera. These days everyone takes pictures on their phones, but if you're old school don't forget to pack your camera!

8. Nursing Pads and Nipple Cream. I didn't need these until after I got home and my milk came in (your baby will be ingesting colostrum for the first 2-5 days after birth) so don't worry about needing these yet. Nipple cream may help with soreness, but the hospital has these items to help you.

Baby's Hospital Bag

Next up, a hospital bag for the baby. This one is a lot less complicated than the mama hospital bag and includes items such as:

1. Onesies (newborn and 3 month since your baby may or may not fit into the newborn size)

2. Special outfit for pictures.

3. Going home outfit (especially if you have guests waiting at your house to meet your baby, it can be fun to dress them in a cute outfit).

4. Socks.

5. Nursing privacy cover (lots of people come in and out of your room at the hospital so pack your nursing cover for privacy).

6. Burp cloths.

7. A special blanket for baby. The hospital provides a baby blanket, but they aren't very soft or cute. I had fun picking a blanket for my daughter and packing it in her hospital bag.

8. A special soft rattle or stuffed animal if you're sentimental, like me. I still have the little grey giraffe I brought with me to the hospital for my daughter.

9. Pacifiers.

Optional items For Baby

1. Aquaphor or Vaseline. If your baby needs these items, the hospital will have them, but you can always bring your own.

2. Chalkboard or cute signs for pictures. I didn't think of this when I had my daughter, but I wish I had! Taking those first few pictures are something you will cherish forever so go ahead…be a little fancy.

3. Diapers. The hospital will provide all the diapers you need! You can even bring some home with you, so save the diapers you bought and got at your baby shower for when you get home.

Dad's Hospital Bag

And last but certainly not least, pack a bag for your partner!
I stocked Will's hospital bag with items such as:

1. Clothes. I made sure to pack him shorts, T-shirts,
   boxers, sweatpants, a hoodie, and some socks. Dad
   needs to be comfortable too!

2. Snacks. I packed all his favorite snacks: candy,
   chips, and beef jerky.

3. Toiletries. I packed him his own set of toiletries, so
   he didn't have to use mine. I included:

   a. Travel sized deodorant
   b. Toothbrush and toothpaste
   c. Travel sized men's body wash, shampoo,
      and conditioner. Trust me, your man will
      want to shower off the trauma of the birthing
      experience too.

4. Chapstick

5. Books or Magazines. Get him a new book if he
   likes to read or a magazine about stuff he likes
   (trucks, dirt bikes, computers, golf, hunting etc.)

If you have other children, it is always a good idea to bring
pictures of them to have out for when they come to meet
the baby. That way, they won't feel like you forgot them.
Also, having a gift to give to your child or children from
the new baby can help them feel special.

Nurse Goody Bags

If you want to score bonus points with your nurses, anesthesiologist, and your doctor, consider making goodie bags! I totally did this and not only were they a blast to make, but the nurses really loved them. Since I was having a girl, I used all pink things. These are the items I put in my goodie bags:

Pink Bath and Body Works Hand Sanitizers
Bubble Gum
Pink Chapstick
Strawberry Special K Bars
A few chocolates

I put all of these in a cute little pink bag with a ribbon and passed them out to all the people who took care of me. It is a simple and inexpensive way to show your nurses and doctors that you appreciate them…and score bonus points so they hook you up with extra stuff!

Birth Plan

Before I start this I just want to say that nothing went according to plan with my labor and birth experience. There are some things even the most neurotic mom (me) just cannot plan for. But, I still believe in having a birth plan and discussing it with your doctor and nurses. This is simply a plan for things you would like to happen and things you are not okay with happening during your labor. You can check Google or Pinterest for help with writing a Birth Plan, so don't worry if you have no idea what to include. Here is my exact Birth Plan for reference:

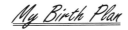

My Name: <u>Lindsey</u>

Baby's Due Date: <u>January 14th</u>

My Doctor: <u>Insert Doctor's Name</u>

Phone Number: <u>Insert Doctor's Phone Number</u>

Primary Support Person: <u>Will</u>
Phone Number: <u>Insert Their Phone Number</u>

Additional Support Person: <u>Melissa</u>
Phone Number: <u>Insert Their Phone Number</u>

<u>During Labor:</u>

- I would like to be able to move around during labor
- I would like to be offered pain management medication and/or an epidural
- I would like the hospital staff to be limited to only my doctor and nurses. Please no students, residents, or interns
- I would like to wear my own clothes as much as possible
- I would like my partner to be with me at all times

During Delivery:

- I would like to be able to push in whatever position is comfortable for me
- I would like to push spontaneously as long as the baby and I are not at risk
- I do NOT want to see the baby crowning or to be offered a mirror. I also do NOT want my partner asked if he would like to see the baby crowning
- I would like a towel or blanket to cover my legs while pushing
- I would like to help catch the baby
- I do NOT want an episiotomy unless it is absolutely necessary

If a C Section is Necessary:

- I would like to stay conscious
- I would like my partner to be with me at all times
- I would like the surgery explained to me as it is happening
- I would like my partner to hold the baby right away. Please check baby while she is with him

Immediately After Delivery:

- I would like the umbilical cord to be cut only after it stops pulsating. Please do NOT cut until I am ready
- I would like to hold the baby immediately after delivery for skin to skin bonding as long as possible. Please check baby while I hold her
- I would like to try and breastfeed right away without assistance
- I would like my partner and/or I to be present during all medical exams and procedures
- Please do NOT give my baby formula or a bottle. I plan to exclusively breastfeed

After Delivery:

- I would like to be alone with my baby for at least 2 hours before visitors are allowed
- I would like all medical procedures explained to me before they are administered
- I would like to be allowed to go home as soon as possible

This is just an example of how you can do your Birth Plan. Unfortunately for me nothing went as I had hoped, and my birth plan went out the window. But, for most women, it is very beneficial to be clear in what you feel is acceptable or not during your labor. Discussing it with your partner or anyone else you plan to have present for the labor is important too, so they can be your voice if anything happens. Remember, it is YOUR labor…no one else's. Never let a doctor, nurse, your mother, or even your partner pressure you into something you aren't comfortable with (unless you or your baby are at risk). YOU are the one having the baby, not them. Period.

The Light at the End of the Tunnel (haha)

Before I went into labor I researched everything I could, asked my mom friends what to expect, and obsessively tried to figure out exactly what was going to happen when my baby came. The truth is, nothing can prepare you for it because every experience will be different. Keep in mind that this is MY story and doesn't mean this will happen to you. Every labor and birth story are different, so don't let this scare you. I don't know a single woman who has a similar birth story to another and yours will be just as unique. But, I want to share my experience with you, so you can understand some of the things no one told me could happen during and after I gave birth.

Did you know that 1/3 of babies born in the United States are delivered via cesarean section (C section)? I certainly didn't, so there was no part of me thinking it could happen to me. I included it in my birth plan more as a formality than anything but never thought about actually going through it myself.

Going into Labor

I assumed my daughter would come early because she did everything early. She dropped about 2 weeks before I had her, causing me to waddle around like a penguin, and was in the birthing position for a week before that. But, she decided she was just too comfy lodged up in my ribcage, and I thought she would never come out. I went to see my doctor on a Monday and at this point, my daughter was four days late. She talked to me about stripping my membranes (ouch) and inducing me on Wednesday if that didn't work. It is very common towards the end of your pregnancy for your doctor to strip your membranes. Let me put this in a way that won't traumatize you completely…basically your doctor will go into your cervix, which is the mouth of the uterus, and will "gently" separate the bag of water from the side of the uterus near the cervix. I'm not going to lie to you, I say "gently" because this procedure is actually quite uncomfortable, and you may bleed a little after. The good news is, this works a lot of the time and can get labor going on its own. It worked for me! My other option was to leave it alone and if the baby hadn't come by Wednesday, they would put a balloon up there to start my dilation…no thank you.

I went home from the doctor, had dinner at about 5:30, and tried to sleep (which was nearly impossible with a child half my size refusing to vacate my womb). At some point I did fall asleep for an hour or two and woke up around 3:31 in the morning to some weird period-like cramping. I was too tired to care so I went back to sleep. I had Braxton Hicks contractions all week, which are basically practice contractions that don't hurt so I ignored it. I woke up again at 5:30 in the morning when Will got up to get ready for work, and that was when it started to get real. My water didn't break, but my contractions were pretty intense. Here's something no one told me about contractions…it may be very difficult to time them. I don't think this is common, but unfortunately for me, I didn't get many breaks between my contractions.

Early in your labor the contractions aren't too bad. They feel like very intense period cramps. I called my nurse and told her I couldn't time my contractions. She told me to head to the hospital in case the baby was going to come fast (I wish). My original plan was to shower, blow dry my hair, listen to some Enya, and cruise to the hospital like a human namaste. NOT. I was so uncomfortable and freaked out that

I skipped the shower, (something I seriously regretted after giving birth) and we headed to the hospital. We called my mom on the way and she met us there. Because my paperwork had already been completed and turned into the hospital during our tour, we were able to be admitted quickly. At this point, you will change into a hospital gown, they will hook you up to some machines, and you may have to wait until a room opens up.

A lot of women will tell you that moving around during pregnancy helps a lot, but for me I couldn't even get up. They moved me to a labor and delivery room and around 1:00 in the afternoon I finally received my epidural. Now, I never wanted to do a natural labor even though it sounded amazing. Letting our bodies do what they are made to do without medical intervention would have been an incredible experience, but I have no shame in the epidural game. I was so miserable at this point that I begged for one.

Let me be clear, whether you chose a natural birth or a medically assisted one...YOU ARE STRONG. You are birthing a child, and nothing about that is easy no matter how you end up doing it. I know plenty of women who had epidurals and wish they hadn't, and I know plenty of women who didn't have an epidural and wished they had! Epidurals are magical when you are in so much pain you feel like you might split in half. It gave me the first real break from pain in almost 8 hours.

After the Epidural

You're probably wondering if the epidural hurts, right? I mean it is a giant needle going into your spine...but let me tell you, I don't even remember it! It's hard to believe someone could actually beg for a needle in their spine, but I did. I remember the whole process, but I don't remember feeling any pain. They have you sign a form, you bend forward, and the anesthesiologist does the rest. Easy peasy. After that, I was able to rest and started to watch some Disney movies to keep me calm. I didn't want to eat because I was nervous about everything going on, but I was able to sip water. Check with your nurses about eating because in the event of an emergency C section, it may be best that you don't eat. Lucky me.

The nurses came in to break my water, which I didn't feel at all, and put a giant "peanut" between my legs. The peanut is a firm, pillow/ball type thing that helps open the pelvic outlet. Never having a baby before, I had no idea what was "normal" and what wasn't. Nurses kept coming into my room and rotating me from one side to the other. When I asked what was going on, they just said that my baby wasn't happy in certain positions and they wanted to try to get her more comfortable. Some time went by, and they decided to put an internal fetal heart monitor on my baby, and they put me on oxygen. The internal monitor is put on the baby's head, so they can better read the heart rate. They also turned off the sound to her monitor, so I couldn't hear anything. I remember feeling nervous about what was going on, but everyone assured me that everything was fine. I was too tired to worry any more than I already was, so I tried to relax. For some reason watching Disney movies was really comforting for me, so I put on Mulan and tried to nap. Something about watching a badass chick save all of China pumped me up.

The Moment Everything Changed

Just as I was about to drift off for a nap, my room was suddenly filled with nurses, and my OB put her hand on my shoulder. Nonchalantly, she told me my baby was in distress and she needed to get her out right away. *Wait, what the what?* I thought to myself as I tried to roll my ginormous belly over to see what was going on. I got stuck half way through and looked like an upside-down turtle. She told me I needed an emergency C section and handed me a form to sign. Instantly, I began shaking so hard my bed was vibrating against the floor. I didn't want to sign the form. I didn't even read it, I just started saying "no, no I can't do this...I don't want to do this". From what I've heard from friends and family, it's very common for all moms to think or say something like this at some point. Giving birth is scary and hard, especially when it's your first baby and you have no idea what to expect! I looked up at my mom and she said, "I know honey. But this is the first of many unselfish things you will do for your baby. You can do this. You must do it for your baby. Everything is going to be all right". Right then and there, I became a mom.

Emergency C Section

Reluctantly, I signed the form. I never read what was on it for fear of going into a full-blown panic attack, but I'm pretty sure it was just going over the risks of the surgery. I was rolled into a freezing cold operating room, and everything was moving so quickly I could barely keep up. I realized that my birth plan was no longer an option, and we just needed to get my daughter out as quickly as possible. Y'all let me just say, if you are a modest person you better prepare yourself to get over any issues you have with being naked in front of people. At this point, my hospital gown was removed, and I was lying buck naked on that table surrounded by doctors and nurses. Also, the number of people who will see your lady business is more than I was comfortable with, but you do what you gotta do for your baby. Just keep this in mind so you can voice anything that makes you uncomfortable ahead of time.

After I got over the fact that I felt like a beached whale ready to be examined by scientists, my anesthesiologist explained that he was going to do something to my epidural and I wouldn't be able to feel anything from the chest down (super). They also tried to strap my arms down and I told them that was not going to happen. I have severe claustrophobia and it was bad enough that I was completely paralyzed. Thank heavens they agreed to let me lay my arms there and didn't strap me down.

The Birth

Everything in that operating room was a blur and I remember feeling a lot of pressure, but no pain. My doctor chit chatted with the nurses about their weekend like they were the ladies from Sex and the City having brunch. Weirdly, this kept me calm because it meant my doctor knew what she was doing and wasn't worried. She was still moving fast, and I had only been on the table for a few minutes. When she said they were going to take the baby out, I didn't think much of it since the process so far had been uneventful. But then the whole table started shaking and my body was rocking back and forth. I looked up at Will, who also had the same look on his face. Bless his heart he tried so hard to contain his horror, so I wouldn't freak out any more than I already was. Then, just like that, they pulled her out. I couldn't see anything except her little foot...and it was blue. I desperately started asking why her foot was blue and why she wasn't crying. I could tell Will was torn between staying with me and going to her when suddenly, she started to cry. We both gasped and smiled at each other.

Immediately After Birth

Hearing your baby cry for the first time is incredible and I felt so relieved that she was okay. Turns out, her umbilical cord was wrapped around her little body twice, and every contraction was squeezing her, causing her heart rate to plummet. Looking back, and knowing my almost 3-year-old very well, it makes complete sense that she was in there doing gymnastics and getting herself tangled and stuck. She still gets herself into crazy situations. Kid's personalities show pretty clearly, even when they're still in your belly.

I was a little upset that I couldn't hold her first, and I had no idea what they were doing to her since I was unable to see her. After a few minutes, Will finally brought her over to me. At first, I was kinda resentful that this little creature had caused me to go through all this hell. I'm totally serious. For a split second I was mad at my newborn. Everyone only ever talks about the overwhelming love they have for their baby and you can judge me all you want, but I am here to be real with you. But, when he moved her closer to me I leaned in and let me tell you... I will never forget her sweet smell. I'm sure you've heard about how good babies smell but when that baby is yours and they're fresh outta the womb, that smell is heavenly. The best way I can describe it is sweet strawberries. Weird right? But it's true. At that exact moment, she smiled at me. I swear on everything that is holy, she actually smiled at me and my heart melted. It was probably just gas, considering she pooped while they were taking her out (she's a classy one), but I like to think it was because she loved me too. It was then that I experienced that overwhelming, unconditional love I had heard so much about. Since I wasn't allowed to move my arms, I was able to nuzzle noses with her (something we still do to this day) and all was right with the world.

Things I Didn't Know About C Sections

Everything after that was even more of a blur. The complete exhaustion set in and I felt like I had been on that table forever. I asked how much longer until I could go to my recovery room, assuming they were almost done, and was told I had another 45 minutes until I was fully sewn up. Here are a few things no one told me about C sections:

1. Your doctor may not be with you through all of this. She came in right before surgery, got the baby out, and bounced. Another doctor was the one who finished closing my incision.

2. Even emergency C sections take a while. They move a lot faster than scheduled C sections, but it's still a major surgery and takes time.

3. They move all your internal organs out of the way. No, they don't actually take your organs out of your body, which is a common misconception, unless they were damaged during surgery. But, they do have to squish them to the side to get to the baby. I asked Will if he could see anything while I was on the table and he said he saw some chunks of what looked like fatty tissue. I remember thinking,

sweet…can they just do a tummy tuck while they're in there? They can't.

4. You may shake uncontrollably. Between the medicine, the stress, and the actual removal of a tiny person, your body may respond by shaking. This scared me at first, but I was reassured that it was normal. It feels like being really cold and shivering, even if you aren't cold.

5. Your doctor will remove the placenta, so you won't have to push it out. One of the benefits of a C section is your doctor can clean and remove everything for you so you can be sure everything is out before being sewn up.

When they were finally done, I was barely able to keep my eyes open. It was like a movie, where you see the person going in and out of consciousness, only that person was me. I don't remember leaving the operating room, but for a short second I came to long enough to see my mom hold my daughter for the first time and she said, "you guys did so good! She's so beautiful!". Then, blackness.

Too Tired to Nurse

I came to again when a nurse was asking me if I wanted to try and nurse. Another thing no one ever told me…you may be too exhausted to even nurse. At the time (and even now if I ever had another baby) I was hellbent on exclusively nursing my baby. I had visions of her coming out, being laid on my chest, and immediately nursing her. But, in that moment where I had nothing left to give, a part of me didn't feel like I was strong enough. To this day, I am so incredibly thankful to Will and my mom for being my voice when I couldn't find mine. This is another reason having a birth plan is so important. Share it with your support system so they can enforce your wants, even if you can't. I remember looking at my mom and telling her I didn't think I could do it. I couldn't even lift my arms to hold her. She told me not to worry and the nurse would hold her for me. Will and the nurse helped her latch, and they moved my arms (while keeping theirs on mine) so I could hold her safely. It was the first time I was able to hold her. I managed to keep my eyes open long enough to see her nursing before I gave into the exhaustion once again.

You Want Me to Do What?

I'm not sure how much time passed since I had fallen asleep, but I rested long enough to be able to lift my arms by myself and keep my eyes open. I got to hold my daughter while they moved me to my recovery room, and I remember shielding her eyes from the bright lights. She was swaddled in a blanket, with a little yellow hat with a pink bow on her head. It was then that the reality of everything that just happened set in. Nothing went according to my birth plan. It's funny looking back because I am such an organized person and I like to control everything. Something like this would happen to me, to teach me that I cannot control or plan for everything. And guess what? I still survived! As scary and difficult as it was, I made it through and was holding my brand-new baby. You can try as hard as you can to prepare yourself for the birth of your child, but stay grounded and know that there is no way to know for sure how everything will go. The best thing you can do is stay calm, let it ride, and never be afraid to make your needs known.

The Road to Recovery

Looking into her eyes I felt so many emotions. I was scared to death that I was responsible for this tiny little person, but I was also filled with so much love and knew I would do whatever it took to keep her safe and healthy. I want you to know that no matter what emotions you feel at this point, they are not only valid, but they are totally normal. Your hormones are going crazy and the trauma of everything will start to catch up to you. You may not feel unconditional love right away, and that's okay! Sometimes it takes a little time to form that bond. You are still a great mom who went through hell to bring your baby into this world.

Once I got to my recovery room, the nurses encouraged me to eat something. At this point, it had been over 27 hours since I had last eaten anything, and I was completely depleted. Most women are ravenous after giving birth, and I always thought I would be too. I totally pictured myself going to town on whatever food I wanted because I earned it! But, I was still so nauseous from the surgery and all the meds that I had to force myself to eat. I finally started to feel better once the epidural began to wear off, and the little bit of food kicked in. For someone with anxiety, being able to feel my legs again made me feel so much better. The only downside to being able to walk again, was the fact that the nurses made me walk to the bathroom. You heard that right… a few hours after major surgery, they told me I needed to get up and walk. The reason for this is to keep everything flowing, prevent blood clots and it actually speeds up the healing process. With a vaginal birth, most women can walk and use the bathroom on their own, even if they had to have stitches. For C section mamas, you will need help getting to the bathroom, so the nurses can clean you, and it may be painful.

You will still have a catheter for about a day after surgery until you can walk better on your own. You will have a ton of fluids in your system, so you'll have to pee more than usual. Since you can't walk much after surgery, they keep it in to help you. So, when I talk about nurses helping you to the bathroom, it is mainly to rinse you off, change your pad, and get you fresh mesh undies.

What Happens After a C Section?

No one ever really talks about what to expect after a C section, but I want to do just that so you can be prepared in case it happens to you. Or if you have a scheduled one. The thing that surprised me the most besides being asked to walk only a few hours after surgery, was the amount of blood I was producing. If you are squeamish, I apologize, but you need to know that you will bleed for some time after childbirth no matter how you do it. According to WebMD, bleeding is how your body gets rid of the extra blood and tissue in your uterus that helped your baby grow. It is totally natural, and the nurses aren't going to care. I was so embarrassed by the mess I was making (not that I could help it), but my nurse acted like it was no big deal. Try to just go with the flow (literally)!

The next thing I didn't know would happen is the nurses will push on your belly every 15 minutes for the first hour after you give birth. This goes for both vaginal deliveries and C sections. I'm not going to lie to you, this is very uncomfortable for C section moms because they push directly on your incision. It is not unbearable, but it will hurt. The reason they do this, is actually for your own good! Once your placenta is removed, all the other vessels are still in there bleeding, and to prevent hemorrhaging the nurses push on your belly to encourage your uterus to contract. Your risk for hemorrhaging is highest during the first hour after you give birth and decreases as time goes on. They are also monitoring how much blood is being produced to make sure you aren't losing too much.

During this time, they may also give you Pitocin to further encourage the uterine contractions and will check your blood pressure. I was losing a little more blood than average, so they started me on an iron supplement to prevent me from becoming anemic. Rest assured that if anything weird starts happening, your nurses will know what to do!

Privacy Please!

Before I went into labor, I knew that there would be a chance for interns to be involved in my labor and recovery. I mean, I've watched Grey's Anatomy enough to know this was a possibility. But, I specifically put on my birth plan that I only wanted my nurses and doctor to take care of me. Some moms have no problem being a part of the learning process, but I wasn't one of them. Being a relatively conservative person, I felt like I had been exposed enough that day and asked for privacy. Unfortunately, I had a nurse who didn't seem to care what my needs were.

When Hospital Staff Doesn't Respect Your Wishes

Let me just say, I was not prepared to go to battle with a total stranger so soon after giving birth. All my labor nurses had been wonderful, and the other recovery nurses were amazing as well, but my night nurse was a different story. Let's be clear, YOU just gave birth. YOU had your body go through enough poking and prodding to have the right to say no to being on display if you aren't comfortable with it. My night nurse kept bringing interns into my room for all my checks. If it had just been blood pressure, medication, and emptying the catheter bag, I wouldn't have had a problem with it. But, my nurse was trying to let her interns watch while she cleaned me and pushed on my belly. She even argued with us when we asked the intern to step out.

I tell you this because I am NOT a confrontational person. If you're similar to me, you may feel bad about asking someone to leave but please, don't. It is your body, your baby, and your experience. I'm no prude, but enough strangers had seen my business that day and I had had enough. Not to mention, this same nurse seemed very bothered by my questions and even ignored our request for my catheter bag to be changed. When you can't go to the bathroom on your own and you need to pee, but your catheter bag is full…it's pretty uncomfortable to say the least. It took her over an hour to actually change it and when she did, she seemed annoyed. If you feel neglected or uncomfortable in any way, ask for a new nurse. I mean it, never be afraid to speak up for yourself. After she stormed out of my room when I declined additional pain medication we finally asked for a new nurse, and it was so much better.

Visitors

I also chose to not let many people visit me after I gave birth because of the trauma. I was experiencing a lot of anxiety, I couldn't shower, and I was pretty nauseous from the medication. I wish I had been able to have friends and family in and out of my room, but I just wasn't up for it. Make the decision for yourself, and don't be afraid to ask for privacy if you need it. This is such a special time for you, your partner, and your baby, so don't feel like you must have people there. They can always visit once you get home and are feeling better.

Homeward Bound

The amount of time you spend in the hospital will depend on how well you are healing and if your doctor feels like you're ready to go home or not. I gave birth on Tuesday and was allowed to go home Thursday. This is actually pretty early for someone to be released, but my OB knew I would heal better at home. I was required to walk on my own down the hallway before she would discharge me, so I did it. It sucked, and I cried the entire time, but I did it. I was so ready to be in my own bed that I would have done jumping jacks had she asked me.

Will brought the car seat into our room so the nurses could help us fit our daughter in it properly. Car seats are intimidating at first so ask for assistance from the hospital staff if you need to. Once she was all buckled in, we signed a bunch of paperwork, packed our stuff, and I was wheeled down to the lobby while Will got the car. I had to continue to take iron supplements and Percocet for pain, so we swung by the pharmacy on the way home. I really didn't want to take any medication, but my doctor pointed out that if I didn't, it would be harder for me to take care of my baby and my healing process would take longer.

I'm not sure how you feel about medication, but if you are anything like me, I don't even like taking Tylenol for a headache. It was hard for me to take such strong pain killers, but I knew my doctor was right. If I was in so much pain that I couldn't even walk, how would I be able to heal and take care of my baby? I relied heavily on ice packs and had to hold a pillow to my stomach whenever I needed to cough or sneeze. That's another thing no one told me about C sections, if you need to cough, sneeze, or laugh, hold a pillow to your stomach because it will hurt like the dickens if you don't. My daughter had a ton of gas one night and was farting more than a truck driver, so I couldn't help but laugh. It felt like I was being cut open all over again, but I just couldn't stop.

Now That You're Home

Being home for the first time with your baby can feel weird. I was so relieved to be home but freaked out at the same time because I felt like I had no idea what I was doing. Thankfully, I had family over to help. Full disclosure…Your body may look like the Pillsbury Doughboy the first week after giving birth. I was a shocked when I looked at myself in the mirror after my first shower because my body was so swollen. My legs and feet were so puffy from all the fluids that I felt like an Oompa Loompa. No one told me I would retain water so viciously, but I am letting you know so you're prepared and don't totally melt down like I did. The good news is all the swelling goes down after about a week so don't panic.

Take advantage of guests being there to help you. I mean it. If they offer to help with laundry or dishes or want to vacuum, please let them do it. They aren't offering out of obligation and they aren't trying to nicely tell you your house is a pigsty. They probably genuinely want to give you a hand. Everyone knows how hard it is to keep your house clean with a new baby so accept their offers and relax while you can. I have a toddler now and wish someone, anyone would come over with a casserole and tackle my massive pile of laundry while I watch Netflix.

When Did I Become a Human Udder?

For the most part, breastfeeding came naturally for me. But, I didn't know that having a C section can prevent your milk from coming in for a few days, so when my baby began cluster feeding, I was a little worried. You will be producing colostrum for the first few days, which is all your baby needs initially. Colostrum is rich in antibodies, so they can live off it until your milk comes in. I was having a little trouble getting my daughter to latch properly (which is very common), so a lactation nurse came in to help while I was still in the hospital. Don't be afraid to ask for help, it does not mean you are doing something wrong! If all moms were able to perfectly breastfeed their baby right away, there wouldn't be any lactation consultants.

Think about it. People actually make a living by helping other women nurse so don't feel like you are a failure if you don't get it right away. The lactation consultant at the hospital helped me try a few different positions until I found the one my daughter liked best. I discovered that my baby was cluster feeding because I wasn't producing enough colostrum, and my milk still hadn't come in after a few days.

How Often Do Babies Eat?

Newborn babies nurse about 8-12 times a day for the first month, and then 7-9 times a day after that according to Kidshealth.org. This means that your baby should go no longer than 2 hours during the day and 4 hours at night between feeds. I know they say never wake a sleeping baby, but in the case of breastfeeding…wake them to eat. Never wait until your baby is crying. Look for signs that your baby is ready to eat, such as rooting (trying to find your boob) and putting their hands in their mouth. With all that being said, try not to worry too much about a feeding schedule until they are older. Babies should be fed on demand unless instructed otherwise by their pediatrician. I used a nursing app to keep track of my daughter's feedings and how long they lasted to show her pediatrician at her checkups. I also used it to keep myself accountable, so I knew when she needed to nurse and could plan accordingly.

It's extremely common for your baby to lose weight after they are born, so you can expect for that to happen. My daughter's pediatrician was a little worried about just how much weight she lost so he had me substitute with formula for a few days to get her weight back up. Naturally, I was devastated but my baby needed the nutrients, so I did it. If you are faced with having to supplement with formula do not give up hope! It doesn't always mean the baby will prefer formula over breastmilk and it doesn't always mean they won't be able to nurse if they take a bottle. I was so worried about her not wanting to nurse, but guess what? She did! After a few days of nursing and supplementing with formula, my milk came in (with a vengeance), and we were able to successfully nurse for 15 months until she self-weened.

If you do choose to use formula and not breastfeed, you may have to try a few different brands before you discover the one your baby likes best. Babies all have different needs, intolerances, and taste preferences so you may have to experiment a little to find the best one.

Nursing can be really tough in the beginning, but if it is something you are passionate about, don't give up! It is not an easy journey by any means, but I can tell you it is SO worth it and your nipples will adjust, I promise. Your breastmilk constantly changes to meet the demands and nutritional needs of your baby. Also, if you or your baby gets sick, you will naturally produce antibodies through your milk to protect and heal your baby. Did you know it can also soothe a diaper rash, treat eczema, and can help heal cuts and scrapes? Breastmilk is amazing!

This Hurts!

If you find yourself with sore, cracked, or bleeding nipples, you can use nipple cream or coconut oil to soothe them. When purchasing a nipple cream from the store or online, check the ingredients and try to purchase a natural one. As I mentioned earlier, even if you wash off before nursing, your baby might still end up ingesting some of it. Better safe than sorry!

Before we move on, I want to talk about clogged ducts and mastitis. You will more than likely face a clogged duct more than once and it may or may not lead to mastitis. I had no idea that this could happen, so when I woke up one day with a large painful lump, I had to Google what to do. I never had any of my clogged ducts turn into mastitis, thank goodness, but I was also very on top of my treatments. Clogged ducts happen when you produce more milk that you can express, and it gets backed up. I overproduced milk like a dairy cow, so I was nursing and pumping throughout the night to try and prevent them from happening. But, I am human, so there were a few nights I was too tired to get up and pump and woke up looking like Pamela Anderson.

What to do

The first thing you should do if you feel a painful swollen lump is to get a hot washcloth and let it sit on your whole breast for a while. I found that the BEST remedy for a clogged duct was letting my baby nurse after the hot compress. Some babies may get frustrated that the milk isn't coming fast enough, but that's a good thing! It causes them to nurse harder, which in turn can loosen the clogged duct! If that still doesn't work, try gentle massage, manual expression, or pumping. There are absolutely no words to describe the relief that comes once the clogged duct is released. Your boob may turn into Niagara Falls but I promise you won't even care.

If you develop a fever, feel achy, or have flu like symptoms, you may be developing mastitis. You should contact your doctor right away, so you can get on antibiotics. Don't worry, the antibiotics will be safe to take while you continue to nurse!

Pumping and Nursing

When my milk finally came in I was producing more than my baby needed. I became engorged and needed to pump in between her feedings. This came in handy because I was able to freeze my milk and use it later. If you decide to stock up on your milk, be sure to always label the bags with dates. Room temperature milk is safe for your baby up to 4 hours. Refrigerated breast milk is safe for up to 3 days, and frozen breast milk is safe for up to 6 months. Always defrost the breast milk in the fridge for about 12 hours or run the frozen milk under warm water. NEVER let it thaw at room temperature. Thawed breast milk is safe for up to 2 hours at room temperature or 24 hours in the fridge. Never refreeze previously frozen milk. Something no one told me about pumping is to never add freshly pumped breast milk to refrigerated breast milk. Always wait until the milk is the same temperature before adding them together. Your thawed milk may smell differently than fresh milk, but don't worry, it should be totally safe for your baby. If it smells really bad though, don't chance it and toss it.

Spit Up

Lastly, I want to warn you about the spit up. You will literally be shocked at how such a small creature can produce that much spit up...but somehow they can. Don't worry, you get used to the smell and will be too tired to care so it's not so bad. Your partner may tell you that you smell like moldy cheese but who cares! Your baby is fed and happy so wear that eau de barfum proudly. Unless you get it in your hair...then yes, girl take a shower. My daughter was spitting up more than I was comfortable with, so I ended up cutting dairy from my diet, and it helped. Our breastmilk flavor can change based off of what we eat, so you may have to adjust your diet if your baby is having issues with spit up. It didn't last long for us, and now she is a total dairy lover! I'm serious don't come near her with a yogurt unless you want to be tackled and robbed. Fair warning.

Hot Mess Express

I mentioned a few times that I ended up with postpartum anxiety, so this chapter will be all about that. I knew that women develop the baby blues or postpartum depression, but I never heard of postpartum anxiety. Not once. I'm not sure why it isn't talked about more or even alongside PP depression but I'm here to address it so you know what to expect.

More Than Anxious

I've always been an anxious person. Even when I was young I liked to have an itinerary, a plan, and know what we were doing each day. I liked routines and hated change. But, I strongly feel like my PP anxiety came from my unexpected C section and the difficult birth of my daughter. I'm not talking about feeling overwhelmed or general new mom jitters. I'm talking full blown irrational anxiety that I subconsciously knew was over the top…but I just couldn't help it.

When I was in the hospital I was afraid to fall asleep. I was convinced that if I fell asleep, I would die. Will had to constantly reassure me that if anything happened while I was sleeping, the monitors would go off and the nurses would help me. Not to mention he was right there with me watching us, but I was still terrified. The nurses wanted to give me anti-anxiety medicine on top of all the other medication and I said no. I was already stressed about the medicine in my system and the potential of getting addicted to them, so I wasn't about to add more. Even when the nurses told me it was safe to take the leg compressions off, I chose to keep them on because I was afraid I would get a blood clot if I did. I barely slept the few days in the hospital and kept my daughter on my chest the entire time to be sure she was breathing too.

Once I got home, the anxiety became less about me and completely about my baby. I read horrifying articles about sudden infant death syndrome (SIDS) and was even anxious to leave her to shower. My family had to beg me to sleep because I was a complete zombie and it was starting to take a toll on my health. I finally agreed to let my mom and grandma watch her, so I could sleep for an hour after feeding her, and I remember lying in bed just listening for any and every noise she made.

Y'all it was BAD. Next level crazy. I also dreaded the evenings because everyone would leave, and Will had to go to bed for work the next day. I was left alone with my baby petrified of sleeping and felt miserable. I spent hours online searching for co-sleeper ideas so I could rest and feel like my baby would be completely safe. I ordered a few options from Amazon, but none of them worked. The only way I could sleep was if I held my daughter and surrounded myself with pillows so she wouldn't fall out of my arms. Obviously, this wasn't a long-term option, and I knew I had to figure something out. My girlfriend from college had twins a few weeks before I had my daughter, and I asked how in the world she was doing it with two babies! That's when she introduced me to the Snuza Hero baby monitor I talked about earlier. I rush ordered it and for the first time in weeks I was able to fall asleep (for an hour) without jolting myself awake from fear.

Co-Sleeping

Even though the Snuza was helping me feel a little more at peace, I still wasn't comfortable letting this tiny baby sleep in a crib by herself on the other side of the house. Not to mention, I was still unable to walk well from my surgery so getting in and out of bed every two hours to nurse just wasn't gonna happen. So, I decided to *gasp* co-sleep with my daughter in my bed. Before you freak out, YES I know it is incredibly risky to let your baby sleep in bed with you, and it increases the chances of SIDS. But, I took every single precaution I could to ensure she was completely safe. You guys…you're talking to a mom who didn't sleep for 3 weeks because she was worried about her baby. I wasn't about to put her in danger.

When it was bedtime, I fed her and put her in her Rock 'n Play right next to my bed. I kept my hand on her chest (and Snuza firmly attached to her diaper) and about an hour later she would wake up to eat. That was when I moved her into bed with me. I kept her on a pillow, with my arm around it and my forehead on her cheek so I would feel her move. I want to be clear that I am not encouraging you to co-sleep unless you do all the research and take all of the necessary precautions. The bed is not a safe place for your baby, so please don't think that because nothing ever happened to me that it can't happen to you. I do, however, encourage you to experiment (safely) and decide for yourself as the mother, where you feel your baby is the safest.

Also, if you decide to co-sleep, be sure your partner knows the risks as well. I am an incredibly light sleeper, so I felt every movement and heard every noise. I also hardly moved at all throughout the night, so I was never afraid of rolling on top of her. But men don't have that motherly instinct and may toss and turn all over the place (insert eye roll). If you choose to bring your baby into bed with you guys, you must be sure that you feel it is the safest option for your baby.

In Conclusion

Having postpartum anxiety doesn't have to only be thought of as a negative thing. In a lot of ways, I feel like it made me a better mom because of the extreme lengths I went to to be sure my baby was safe. It also drove me to research the crap out of EVERYTHING so I was always prepared for the apocalypse. If you feel off after you give birth, just know you are not alone. PP depression and anxiety are very common and can happen to anyone. Reach out for help, talk to your support system, and speak to your doctor if you feel like you need further assistance. My postpartum anxiety eased up a lot as my daughter got older, and the risk of SIDS was drastically reduced (around 6 months-1 year). You will get through this season so even if it feels hard, try to focus on all the memories and bonding time with your newborn because it goes so fast.

What is Happening?

Something that definitely didn't help with my postpartum anxiety was the fact that newborns do some weird ass stuff when they're first born. NO ONE told me my baby would scare the crap out of me on the regular, so let me share with you some things newborns do that are totally normal but may freak you out.

1. They may look cross-eyed. This can last until they are about 4 months old and it happens because babies have to learn how to make their eyes work together. The muscles that control your baby's eyes are developing so don't worry too much. If your baby is constantly cross-eyed, seems to have vision problems, or is older than 4 months old and is still cross-eyed, then check with their pediatrician to be sure everything is okay.

2. Sleeping with their eyes open. As if being cross-eyed wasn't bad enough, your baby may also sleep with their eyes open! No one really knows why it happens, but it is totally normal in babies under a year old. If you're worried, you can gently stroke them closed.

3. Cradle cap. According to Mayo Clinic, cradle cap causes crusty or oily scaly patches on a baby's scalp. No one knows what causes it, but one contributing factor may be hormones that pass from the mother to the baby before birth. These hormones can cause too much production of oil (sebum) in the oil glands and hair follicles. It may look weird, but I assure you it isn't painful or itchy. When my daughter developed it, I put pure coconut

oil on her scalp, massaged it in, let it sit for 15 minutes, and then used a soft brush from her grooming kit to buff it off. I cannot tell you how amazingly this worked! It was gross, but it cleared it up within a few days!

4. Startling themselves awake. This probably scared me more than anything else my daughter did those first few weeks home. She would be sleeping soundly and then all of a sudden, she would throw her hands in the air and jump! She literally startled herself awake. This, in turn, made me jump too. Most times, she went right back to sleep but a few times it was bad enough to scare her and make her cry. When I frantically began researching what on earth was going on, I found out that it was actually a good thing! Babies nervous systems are developing, and this is a natural reaction to what feels like falling for them. It's scary, yes, but it's normal and means their reflexes are reacting the way they should be. Swaddling is the best way to prevent this from happening, but it still may happen no matter what you do to prevent it.

5. My daughter turned blue after her first bath. Thank the Lord above I had my mom and my grandmother with me when this happened because I about lost my mind. Newborn babies have a hard time regulating their body temperatures, so it is totally common for their hands and feet to turn a little blue when they get chilly. They may even shiver. The best way to prevent this is to have a warm towel ready to go so you can wrap them in it right after their bath. You should worry if your baby's torso is also blue, as this can mean they aren't getting enough oxygen.

6. Pulsing head and soft spots. Your baby will have two soft spots on their head when they are born, one on the top and one in the back. The reason for this is your baby's head bones are somewhat soft and mostly connected by tissue when they are in the womb. This allows for your baby's head to fit through the birth canal...hence the cone shaped head after a vaginal birth. As your baby gets older, the bones will fuse together, and the soft spots will close. In the meantime, the gaps allow for the rapid brain and skull growth. Be gentle with these areas and never push on them. Your pediatrician will check them at all of your visits, but if you ever see them sunken in it could mean a serious health problem or dehydration. They will often pulsate too, so don't freak out! The one in the back should close around 4 months old, and the top one should close between 9-18 months or age 2 at the very latest.

7. Grunting, snorting, and strange breathing patterns. Babies make all sorts of noises...mostly cute, but some are downright weird. As long as your baby is healthy and doesn't have a cold, grunting and snorting are totally normal. Their little nostrils can get congested easily so if it's bad, try some saline drops. As far as the breathing patterns go, it's normal for them to pause, then take a few rapid breaths. The main reason for this is their respiratory systems are immature and still developing. Keep in mind that weird breathing patterns are VERY different from not breathing or struggling to breathe. If you feel in any way that your baby is struggling to breathe, call for help.

The Royal Treatment

Another way I got my PP anxiety under control was…you guessed it…establishing a routine with my baby. As you know by now, I'm very organized. I like to plan and thrived on a routine as a child. I figured that was a brilliant way to keep things under control and remove the additional anxiety I was facing.

Bedtime Routine

The first thing I did was establish a bedtime routine. I found it a little difficult to stick to a naptime routine at first because her naps were a little all over the place when she was little. That changed as she got older and I did get her naps down to a science. I was able to implement a successful bedtime routine when she was 3 months old. You may have to test out a few things to figure out what works for your baby, but I learned that a lot of babies respond very well to a similar pattern. Walk outside, playtime, bath, massage, feed, bed.

I live in Arizona and had my daughter in January, so thankfully it was cool enough to take my daughter on walks at night. It takes about 6 weeks to recover from a C section, so I was able to start taking her on walks by myself around 2 months old. If it's too hot to do a walk, try some short outside time to let your baby see the trees, hear the birds and look at the flowers. It's very soothing to be outside, even for babies. It started to get dark around 6:00, so after our walk I would let her do some tummy time and play with her on her play mat. When she started to get fussy, I would give her a warm bath followed by a massage. You can look online to learn how to give your baby a massage because it is hard to explain without visuals. I highly recommend it though. Think about how relaxed you are after a massage! Same goes for your baby. I used pure coconut oil, and gently rubbed her little body until she was sleepy. Finally, I would nurse her until she fell asleep and bada-bing bada-boom…bedtime routine complete!

If it sounds too good to be true, I assure you it's not. Once I realized how quickly and easily this worked I began sharing it with all of my new mom friends. They couldn't believe how well it worked for them too! Babies, toddlers, and children all need some sort of structure and routine in their lives because it gives them a sense of stability, so why not start as soon as possible? Give it a try and adjust as needed, but after a few days your baby's body will adjust to the new schedule and be sleepy right on time!

A major issue in the beginning with newborns is they can get their days and night mixed up. You gotta cut the tiny people some slack though because in their defense they were in a dark womb up until they were born. You can imagine how much of a change that is for them. Let your newborn nap when they want to, but it is also a good idea to let them be outside and play with them during the day. That way, they will become accustomed to being awake while it's light out. At night, keep everything calm, quiet, and dark so they can learn that is when they sleep. Even when they wake up to nurse, try to keep things as quiet and dark as possible so they don't think it's time to wake up.

Brave New World

So now that you're breastfeeding like a boss, you've established a successful bedtime routine, and are finally getting the hang of this motherhood thing, it's time to venture out into the world... by yourself... for the first time...with a baby. I will be honest here, I was so freaked out thinking about being alone with my daughter in public for the first time, but I needed to get off of house arrest. I have a Target about 5 minutes from my house and was having major withdrawals, so I decided that would be a good place to go!

Target With a Baby

I showered (which I only did a few times a week if I was lucky), threw on some tinted moisturizer and mascara, made sure my diaper bag was fully stocked, ate a snack, fed my baby, and loaded her in the car. Now, to be fair I had left the house a few times before this for doctor and pediatrician appointments, but I always had someone with me because I wasn't allowed to drive on pain killers. This was the very first trip I was taking with just the two of us, (Target is still our favorite place to go together) and I was nervous.

After I made sure she was nice and full, I stuffed some nursing pads in my bra and headed for the car! I remember thinking, huh, look at all these people out here with their lives. When you're trapped in a house for weeks on end it's easy to forget there is an entire world out there with other people still going about their business. I felt so relieved to rejoin the human race that all my fears went away. I popped her car seat out and into a shopping cart and headed inside.

The air hit my face as I walked in and the lovely Target smell filled all of my senses. *Dang it feels good to be back!* I thought to myself as I browsed the nail polish and makeup aisles. My daughter was asleep, so it was really nice to have a little break.

A ton of people approached me, which caught me completely off guard, because they wanted to take a peek at my baby. I felt a little exposed, and since I was still battling with my anxiety, I started to panic a little. I didn't want anyone touching or even breathing near my baby, so I decided to hide out in the baby section with the other moms. Total strangers may approach you and try to touch your baby, and I want you to know that it is completely okay to politely tell them to back off. Or you can buy a car seat cover that will give your baby complete privacy with a little window where you can peak in and see them. I didn't know they existed when I had my daughter, but man I wish I had. Every time anyone even looked like they were coming towards me, I avoided eye contact and went another direction. Maybe I'm nuts, I don't know, but I just didn't want my tiny baby exposed to anything germy or weird. Just be prepared for people to come outta the woodwork to stare at your baby.

When I was safely in the baby section, I grabbed some cute headbands and got totally carried away in the clearance section (every time Target, every time). I lost track of time, and when my daughter woke up all hell broke loose. It was time to feed her, and I had a whole cart full of stuff I needed to pay for. She was hysterically crying, and I felt like the entire store was looking at me. I immediately picked her up and tried to comfort her but knew there was no way I could buy my items and make it home before feeding her. So, I made a decision. I could either abandon my cart, run to my car, and drive 100 mph to get home, or I could buy my stuff and nurse her in public.

I decided to bite the bullet and nurse her in public. I mean, it was bound to happen at some point right? Might as well get it over with! I paid for my items (with her still fussing) and went to my car. I threw the bags in the trunk and climbed in the backseat with her. Right then and there, in the Target parking lot, I nursed my baby. People were walking by, so I covered up with her blanket and it actually wasn't too bad! I ended up having to nurse her in the car a few times and it was never a big deal. Thank heavens for nursing bras with easy access! We should have the right to feed our babies whenever and wherever we need to. I am all for nursing in public and got pretty comfortable doing it. It's a blessing because it really frees you up from having to rush home to nurse. Do what works for you, mama. You'll figure it out!

Go Forth and Be Amazing

I think I covered everything I didn't know could happen during pregnancy, childbirth, breastfeeding, and life with a newborn but of course I am still a mom and probably forgot some stuff too. We are all just doing our best, aren't we? There is no rule book on how to do this motherhood thing the "right" way so you are just going to have to figure out how to do things your way. We all have mother's intuition, so listen to her and let her guide you. Even when she's being a psycho Sally.

I want to reiterate that asking for help at any point along the way does not make you a bad mom. It makes you a better mom because you are recognizing you need help and are taking the steps necessary to correct something you are struggling with. This will always benefit you and your baby in the end so reach out and find a support system.
Being a mother is the hardest job in the world, so be gentle on yourself. Be sure to find time to do things you enjoy, even if it's just scrolling Pinterest while you nurse your baby or painting your toes in between naps. You are the glue that holds everything together, so make self-care a priority for the sake of everyone who depends on you. You are worth it!

Made in the USA
Middletown, DE
01 March 2023